Management and Practice in Emergency Nursing

Management and Practice in Emergency Nursing

Edited by
BOB WRIGHT
Senior Charge Nurse
Accident and Emergency Department
Leeds General Infirmary

London
CHAPMAN AND HALL

First published in 1988 by
Chapman and Hall Ltd
11 New Fetter Lane, London EC4P 4EE

© 1988 Bob Wright

Typeset in Times by Mayhew Typesetting Ltd
Printed in Great Britain by
St Edmundsbury Press Ltd
Bury St Edmunds, Suffolk

ISBN 0 412 28460 X

British Library Cataloguing in Publication Data

Management and practice in emergency
nursing.
  1. Medicine. Emergency treatment. Nursing
  I. Wright, Bob, 1943–
  610.73'61

  ISBN 0–412–28460–X

Contents

Contributors

Joseph Blansfield RN, MS, CEN
Clinical Nurse Specialist, Emergency Department, Boston City Hospital, Boston, Massachusetts, USA.

Peter Blythin RGN, RMN, Dip Nursing, CANS
Deputy Director of Nursing Services, North Staffordshire Royal Infirmary, Stoke-on-Trent, England.

Dianne M. Danis RN, MS, CEN
Former Assistant Director of Nursing, Adult and Paediatrics Emergency Department, Boston City Hospital, Boston, Massachusetts, USA.

Gary J. Jones SRN, OND, Dip Nursing REMT, FETC
Head of Accident and Emergency Nursing Services, Orsett and Basildon Hospitals, Basildon and Thurrock Health Authority, England.

Susan McGuinness FCJ, RGN, RSCN
Staff Nurse / Bereavement Counsellor, Accident and Emergency Department, Hope Hospital, Salford, England.

Jill Milnthorpe RGN
Nurse Manager of Emergency Services, Milton Keynes District Hospital, Milton Keynes, England.

Kate O'Hanlon MBE, RGN, RM
Senior Sister, Accident and Emergency Department, Royal Victoria Hospital, Belfast, Northern Ireland.

Hilary Wareing RGN, RM, HV Certificate
Research and Liaison Health Visitor, Accident and Emergency Department, Leeds General Infirmary, Leeds, England.

Bob Wright SRN, RMN, Certificate in Counselling
Senior Charge Nurse, Accident and Emergency Department, Leeds General Infirmary, Leeds, England.

Foreword

I am delighted to be asked to write the Foreword for *Management and Practice in Emergency Nursing.*

More than any other nursing speciality Accident and Emergency work reflects change in society because it is the casualties of social upheaval, imbalance and inequality that you face every day.

Here, unfortunately, A and E staff are confronted on a regular basis with child abuse, family violence, the result of terrorist activities, social violence, motor car accidents, personal loss of loved ones, the frustrations and aggression of life. Sometimes, though, some pleasant and funny episodes do occur but all too infrequently to become the norm.

My own experience of A and E nursing is very limited; in fact, it goes back to the days of the Department being linked with Orthopaedics and being called 'Casualty'. It could, though, appear that in this day and age the wheel is turning full circle and moves have been made in the last reorganization to link the two new distinct specialities again. This proposal was met with lots of protest from A and E staff which appears to have been defused. The arguments stemmed mainly from the fact that orthopaedics and A and E are two quite difficult specialities of care and skills and as such must be seen as autonomous.

Although my 'hands on' experience in this field is limited, I have over recent years had a great deal of contact with A and E nurses and I feel very strongly that A and E nurses have had a major part to play in advancing and highlighting the differences and difficulties that are experienced in this front-line Department. The only shadow over my observations is that the committed are but a few compared with the overall number of nurses working within A and E. Nurses being nurses have been reluctant to join the forward thinking and have, to a degree, jeopardized their cause.

The pleasure I found in this book is the commitment of the authors to improving not only the service to patients but the fulfilment of and standards for nurses as well.

All authors have had practical experience in implementing their particular concepts and have suffered the rejection and disappointments connected with advancing skills and practice, only to pick themselves up, evaluate and continue undeterred. I remember a particular incident in which Bob Wright was speaking to a group of A and E nurses about encountering and dealing with violence. His reception was, to put it mildly, hostile; undaunted, however, he continued, and through perseverance and commitment ideas are being changed. I now frequently hear of hospitals training staff in communication skills and how to identify problems and defuse them before major incidents arise.

This book identifies areas that not so many years ago were taboo — nurses commissioning new departments, working on an equal footing with other care workers, involved in quality assurance, making decisions about priorities of care, and leading the way in new approaches to A and E care.

My hope is that this book will be read and discussed further by nurses. Those who are still back in 'Casualty' will think and decide that now is the time to relook, rethink and, hopefully, review their concepts and practices. Patients need nurses. Let us state our potential and influence ideas.

Susan E. Russell
Professional Development Officer
Royal College of Nursing

Editor's Introduction

The work of the emergency nurse is diverse and full of extremes. It ranges from the fingertip injury to the patient with multiple injuries. Patients are not always comfortable in the role of patient. They are taken rapidly from their work, their home, their recreation, and so often quickly joined by their families who want them home and have strong emotional needs. We are confronted with a unique and often highly emotionally charged situation.

A nurse may have to move from a well-ordered, clean clinical setting to work in the tangled wreckage of a multiple accident. The patient may be passive and compliant or distressed and aggressive — life and death, wealth, happiness, misery and poverty are all there. The nurse will be presented with the mundane, the complicated and the results of political whims and policies. Where do we begin to educate the nurse for all this? Fortunately, we have a base on which to build.

Emergency nurses are better motivated than many of their peers in seeking re-education and this trend is demonstrated internationally. Professional organizations for emergency nurses are well-supported and thriving. On meeting many nurses from this field internationally at recent conferences I quickly felt a camaraderie and realized that this work has few or no national boundaries. I have heard nurses from rural Mexico, the UK, US, bustling cities and strife-torn countries share experiences. We have much to teach each other on a practical and professional level and we have much in common. These nurses were eager to share experiences, to confront the calm, the chaos and the ambiguity and to encounter the individual. The ability to encounter each patient, a unique individual with any of a diversity of conditions, and be part of the overall management of the Department takes special skills and commitment.

This book is for you. It is not just another textbook for the emergency nurse. It will not deal with a long list of clinical conditions. It explores aspects of the work and the individual that merit more of our thought and innovation. It will take you out to the tangled wreckage of the road accident, guide you through the planning of your Department and explore clinical aspects of evaluation and priorities. The management of disaster, death and aggression sounds like a tall order, but you will find examples of experience and innovation in these areas, putting structure into chaos.

The importance of children's needs and the role for nurses in liaising with other departments is discussed.

Last but not least on my list of priorities, come our needs as nurses: our education and personal development. I know each contributor and have heard them all speak about their work. They all work with their specialist subject and are keen to share their expertise with you. The nursing knowledge that is here is for real.

I commend their work to you and hope you experience some of their enthusiasm and the excitement as well as the difficulties of this work, and that you feel more effective in your personal and professional lives.

1

The Nurse's Role in Planning and Commissioning an Accident and Emergency Department

Jill Milnthorpe

'Lists, lists and more d . . . d lists.' Ask any Accident and Emergency nurse what improvements he or she would make to the department and the list will be varied and endless. Each person will have different ideas and this is rightly so, as each department serves a different community and has different needs. The nurse's view will be overlaid by the views of consultants, management, accountants and architects. Each will see or desire different features and it is the job of the planning and commissioning team to marry all these into a workable department that serves the purpose for which it is designed.

Capital schemes, comprising totally new departments, do not occur very often. Modification or improvement of existing departments to meet increased need is more usual, but the same principles apply and can be utilized for smaller schemes.

The role of the nurse member of the planning team is to represent the nursing point of view. He or she may be the only member of the team with the specific working knowledge of how a department carries out its day-to-day function. She will need to translate this into terms that the architect can understand, so that he can provide working drawings for the builder to translate into the finished shell.

Already the complexities of the project begin to emerge and we realize that all the jobs of the people concerned will overlap. The architect has to work within the confines of both the capital funding and the current DHSS building regulations (CAPRICODE) as well as any local building regulations; for example, in a new town there may be specific requirements to meet the overall planning system, whereas in a different situation the architect may have to 'match' existing buildings.

None of this is done in isolation. The nurse planner will work with the planning team but should, where a change or modification is being carried out to an existing department, also seek the views of nursing staff prior to and during all the phases of planning. She will also visit other units to seek information. The department may be planned with a future project to be added within a given time. This will also affect the way the initial project is planned and managed. The nurse planner will need to understand the working drawings of what is to be included in the future project and its operational systems. Consultation with all other disciplines who may be affected by the initial or future planned project is also necessary.

The nurse planner will also need to have information about equipment so that she can advise the planning team with regard to its functional performance, its cost and whether the item is essential or desirable. It is important in any scheme to differentiate between the latter two. Items that are essential would include such things as patient trollies, electrocardiograph machines and resuscitation equipment. Desirable items may be monitors for each cubicle or other specialist equipment.

The complete commissioning team works to exact terms of reference, which are set with the objective of bringing each new project to the state of readiness for operational use. The nurse planner is an essential part of this team.

1.1 OPERATIONAL SYSTEMS

The operational policy of a new department will have been drawn up by the commissioning team and its advisers. An operational system is the translation of these policies into practice, so that the financial guidelines, equipment requirements, design solutions and staffing requirements fulfil the intention of the policy. The operational policy is a basic outline only and it is the operational system that allows a degree of flexibility in the running of the department. It is these systems that will determine which equipment is bought, how many staff are employed, the level of service to be provided and the subsequent revenue costs to the organization.

By the nature of the work done in Accident and Emergency Departments, all other departments within the hospital impinge on it, and at times (e.g. during major incidents), it impinges on them.

However, although consultation and communication among these departments is essential, it is important that the prime user — the patient — is kept in mind. When everyone is trying to obtain the best for his or her discipline, it is very easy for the patient to be overlooked. This is again where the role of the nurse planner is paramount. She can act as the patient's advocate when decisions such as relatives' rooms, patient movement and sub-pharmacies are discussed and written into the operational system.

A working group is usually set up to draw up operational systems. Not all members will attend every meeting, but their decisions will be recorded and written into the operational systems manual. This will then provide a logical system for putting the policy into action.

Typical operational systems manuals for an Accident and Emergency Department will include:

1. A brief statement of the operational policy.
2. The services to be provided, including other specialist functions such as radiographic service and clinics; normal hours of work; on-call and emergency arrangements; and predicted workload.
3. Organizational structure, which will show lines of accountability within the department and, where appropriate, within the hospital.
4. Costed staffing structure, which will show the proposed grading and number of staff for each group working within the department, including such variables as units of medical time (UMTs) for medical staff, special duty payments (nursing), bonus payments (porters, domestic) and shift differential (porters, clerical). It will take into account the number of staff to be deployed in each shift, together with a built-in differential to allow for annual leave.
5. Budgetry arrangements. Traditionally, the head of the Nursing Department has held the nursing budget; medical and surgical supplies have been held on a central budget and capital equipment has been brought through the administration. This system has gradually changed and departmental budgets are now the norm. The operational system manual should set out clearly who is to be budget-holder and exactly what this budget is expected to cover. It is worth spending time at the planning stage to decide this, as it prevents problems at a later stage when everyone decides that his pet piece of equipment is absolutely essential.
6. Departmental records system, which define how records are

obtained, recorded and stored. The Korner recommendations (1982) and codings should be incorporated into any records and where the project is a modification of an existing department, this may be the opportunity to introduce change. It is more usual nowadays for computers to be used to record patient attendance, and manual records to be microfiched for storage. The recommendations of the Data Protection Act (1984) should be adhered to. This section of the planning system must contain details for security of information.

7. Relationships with other departments and services. Relationships depend on communication and personality rather than the written word. However large the organization, it is always worthwhile to use the personal touch and discuss with either heads of departments or contract service managers those services that they will provide to the department. Having said this, it is then essential that the conclusions reached are recorded for clarity and future reference, for example, services to be provided by the domestic department, accountability and responsibility of portering staff.

8. Departmental procedures, which define and summarize the way the department will be run. As these affect in part the specification of equipment to be either built in or bought, it is again important that time is spent on them. At first glance it may be felt that they are self-explanatory, but it is always useful to have a checklist as they will give an indication of financial consequences.

Staffing

Medical organization
Nursing organization
Clerical staff
Portering staff
Overnight beds
Cinics
Theatre
Plaster room
Facilities for children

Equipment

Resuscitation facilities
Major accident
Major and minor treatments
Needs for specical areas,
   e.g. mines, mountains

Documentation

Admission procedures
Transfer to specialist units
Patients' property

General Considerations

Ambulance arrival
Police liaison
Paediatric liaison

Documentation	**General Considerations**
Records procedures	Geriatric liaison
Patients brought in dead	Social services liaison
	Community service liaison
	Local voluntary support services,
	e.g. Samaritans, battered
	wives refuge
	Car parking for patients
	Car parking for staff

9. Management Systems. This cross-references with other departments that could also serve the Accident Department.

This list is not totally definitive, nor should it be regarded as such. Manuals are the bones of the project. They give direction and aims, both for the commissioning team and for those who come after, so that the initial thoughts of the planners become reality.

1.2 ACTIVITY DATA SHEETS

Activity data sheets are not part of the operational systems manual, but complement it. Both are necessary to a planning project, but there is, again, no single correct way of compiling these. By drawing up the operational system, we may identify what the needs of the new project are; by looking at other departments and their success or failure, we may decide how to use the space available prior to working out the operational system. Modification of an existing department may start with activity data sheets.

For the nurse planner carrying out a project for the first time, it is useful to look at data sheets from previous projects. These, together with the previously identified essential and/or desirable items, will provide a base from which to work out the use and content of each room or area. Some regions will have their own sheets which are almost standard, especially if 'nucleus' type building has taken place. Most are based on the DHSS Activity Data Book, which provides up-to-date specifications for the type of activity likely to be carried out in that area. This may be one of the areas where the nurse planner's working knowledge is best utilized. Diplomatic negotiation is sometimes needed to convince members of the design team that what is good on paper would be impractical and would not suit local conditions.

The top sheet on an activity data schedule outlines the activity that will be carried out in that room, the equipment that will be located there and necessary environmental conditions. It will show the wall and floor finishes. This sheet is known as the A sheet. The following B sheets expand and explain the A sheet in detail. These are divided into groups, showing those services and spaces that are supplied and fitted by the builder, those supplied by the Health Authority and fitted by the builder, those supplied and fitted by the Health Authority after handover of the building, and those that have no space implications for the builder but which are on departmental equipment lists. Examples of departmental equipment are engineering terminal outlets, lighting or medical gases, sphygmomanometer, patient and dressing trollies.

1.3 ESSENTIAL AND DESIRABLE AREAS OF AN ACCIDENT DEPARTMENT

Accident and Emergency has emerged as a speciality in its own right over the last 20 years. Despite this, many departments are still tied to the orthopaedic service of the hospital. The inception of a new department or modification of an existing one may provide an opportunity to rethink this policy of dual use. Emergency orthopaedic work provides a small part of any department's function today. The progress within the speciality of orthopaedic service has also meant that more diagnostic and reconstructive work is done, so it makes sense to use the facilities of the Out-patients Department rather than the Accident Department.

For those departments providing a Major Incident service, it is essential that full facilities for storage of all 'call-out' equipment are provided. Staff changing rooms with shower facilities are also considered essential. All Accident and Emergency nurses who have had to finish a shift wearing a theatre gown or who have had to traverse the length of a busy hospital corridor covered in vomit or washout fluid would agree!

Night facilities for medical staff are also essential. If the medical staffing is such that a night shift cover cannot be provided, then it is essential that a sleeping facility is provided within the department.

Desirable features will depend on the workload area served and facilities that may be already available and can be modified.

One of the most essential features for any modern Accident Unit, assuming that full resuscitation facilities have already been provided, is the staff rest room. Perhaps 'rest room' is a misnomer, as the opportunity for rest is infrequent. It is, however, necessary to provide such a room, removed from the patient area but within the department, where staff can take time out. Accident and Emergency nursing can be very stressful. It deals with the immediate — the injured child, the sudden death, the violent or verbally abusive. It is necessary to provide a place to withdraw to, to make a cup of coffee, regain composure, cool off and prepare to start again. This room can also be used for formal teaching and group or individual counselling. It must be recognized that the needs of the staff as well as patients should be served. This highlights another role for the nurse planner: the staff advocate.

1.4 MODERN CONCEPTS OF AN ACCIDENT UNIT

The emergence of the speciality of Accident and Emergency has already been described. Along with this have come changes in the way the Accident Department is viewed by its staff and patients. Technology and advances in medical science have also imposed change. Change should not be difficult for the Accident nurse to accept; after all, it is the bread and butter of her everyday life. A new department, or changes in an existing one, will allow change to occur. The nurse planner may or may not have in-depth knowledge of the workings of an Accident Unit and should seek advice from those who have.

It is not proposed to deal with all items in depth, as this will be done in other chapters, but rather to outline those areas in which change can be considered.

1.4.1 Reception area

This area should be large enough for the clientele it is expected to serve, but not so large as to be impersonal and threatening. It should be designed so that the nursing staff are in visual contact with it. Colours should be bright and pleasing. There should be a children's waiting area, with child-size chairs, toys and, if possible, a nursery nurse to supervise the area. Video films can be provided to educate and to offer a distraction.

An area adjacent to reception should be provided for nurse triage. If the department is new, it will probably have a computer terminal. This will facilitate registration, printing of in-patient notes and appointments. The registration area and glass doors should ideally be constructed of reinforced glass. It is a sad reflection of today's society that hospital staff now need protection against violence. The triage desk would ideally be situated so that the triage nurse could retreat to the registration area if necessary.

Violence towards staff and other patients requires that security systems need to be built into Accident Departments. Ideally, there should be at least two sorts of systems, so that there is a 'fail-safe' cover. Panic buttons should be in direct contact with the switchboard, with a specific written response action to be carried out, for example, instructions to phone police and porters. Departmental cover call systems and video recording cameras all need to be considered. The presence of a security officer during high-risk periods may be a deterrent. A porter should always be working within the department. It should also be possible to work out a rota between medical and nursing staff so that 'all female' groups are never left alone in the department.

It is always worth compartmentalizing the department so that the various areas can be kept separate, as necessary.

The minor treatment area should be adjacent to the waiting area, allowing easy access for patients.

There should be a separate ambulance entrance that does not connect with the general waiting area. Adjacent to this should be the resuscitation facility. The size of this will depend on the area served, but it should have flexibility. It should be able to take at least two patients, with room for another as required. In a major capital project, the equipment for this room should match others within the project, for example, in theatres or intensive care. If the defibrillator, monitors, and so on are all identical, it causes less confusion for short-term medical staff and also allows servicing on a contract basis to be arranged.

The equipment list for the resuscitation room is often made the task of a medical member of staff. I believe it is for the nurse planner, again, to put forward the nursing point of view. Equipment should be wall-mounted on a rail system wherever possible and be readily accessible.

1.4.2 Acute treatment area

This is best located near the resuscitation facility and ambulance entrance. There are many different thoughts on the equipping of cubicles for the acutely ill patient. This author has seen some that are so full of equipment there was hardly room to treat the patient. It is probably better to keep basic equipment in each room and all treatment facilities on a central console. Each cubicle should have a panic button as well as a communication facility. It is worth considering having at least two rooms with solid doors, as opposed to curtains, for containing patients who are violent. Lights should be flush-fitting and equipment should not be wall-mounted, but easily removable. Depending on the proposed usage of the department, it may be worth considering whether separate facilities should be provided for gynaecological examination, ophthalmic examination or isolation.

There should be a facility in which an area can be cordoned off for radiation or chemical decontamination. This could include the isolation area, or one that is in general use, with decontamination equipment stored nearby. A shower or bathroom facility for patients is useful, but it must be remembered that noxious substances should not be allowed into the general sewage system.

(a) Plaster room facility

This is one of the busiest parts of any Accident and Emergency Department. It is important to provide a sub-waiting area, and again, video health education can be used to advantage. Plenty of working space is required so that beds can easily be brought into the room, and with modern splintage materials there should also be facilities for construction of plasterzote splints and so on. The use of this room should also be clearly defined. As with all space in Accident and Emergency Departments, it is often expected to absorb all those patient services that cannot be fitted in elsewhere in the hospital. Appliance measuring and fitting is not part of an Accident Department facility and should be properly provided for in the Out-patients Department.

(b) *Minor procedures theatre*

This, again, can be misused. An Accident Department is not the place for removal of lumps and bumps and planned minor surgery. The minor procedures theatres should be set up and equipped to deal with accidents and emergencies as they occur. It should be able to cope with anything except major surgery.

1.5 COMMISSIONING

However well-planned any programme is, the planning team is always in the hands of the builders and suppliers. Large capital schemes usually have a target date for handover of the building, but this may have to be extended if the contractor meets unexpected problems. Changes of specification during the building programme may occur which delay the handover and have implications for all the stages that follow.

The nurse planner and/or the nurse member of the commissioning team will need to be aware of any delays in the handover, but can do little to influence them. The main problem will be to co-ordinate the equipment delivery so that it arrives in the right place at the right time. If there is a long delay in the handover, it may not be possible to delay accepting supplies, so local storage facilities with adequate security will have to be arranged. The possibility of this happening should always be kept in mind and contingency plans should be made prior to ordering. This will prevent even further delays when the building is eventually handed over.

The supplies officer has the responsibility for the purchase, delivery, inspection and storage of all new equipment. He will work to the specifications on the Activity Data B sheet, but will need to know the type, model and catalogue number of specific equipment required. His job is to keep within the budget allowed for each item, but he does not and cannot have specific knowledge of how it is used. A competent nurse planner / commissioning nurse will be able to advise the supplies officer not only of the requirements but also of the timing of delivery, so that large items and those that require special installation are delivered at the right time. It would be useless to have delivery of medical and surgical consumables before trolleys; it would be equally silly to receive large stocks of linen before the cleaning has been carried out. The department head should be in post at the time of handover. Together with the commissioning nurse, she will draw up lists for systematic phasing-in of the department.

One of the first tasks will be to carry out an inspection for snags. This identifies any missing items that the contractor must complete or rectify before the liability period is over. This will be followed by a 'Design in Use' period of up to a year after handover, when the users of the department will have identified any defects or problems for which the contractor can be held responsible. As in a private dwelling, it is not worth calling in the contractor for every minor fault as it arises, but a log book should be kept so that at the end of the 'Design in Use' period they can be rectified. Obviously, major problems such as plumbing or air conditioning should be reported immediately.

Cleaning of all the areas must be carried out prior to delivery of furnishings and equipment. The areas used for treatment will need to be swabbed and the swabs cultured by the Pathology Department for bacteriological clearance prior to occupation.

Using the Activity Data B specifications, the equipment and furniture for each room should be checked off and labelled with the room number. This will immediately identify those items that are missing or still awaiting delivery. The supplies officer should chase suppliers for these items; it can be totally confusing for all concerned, not least of all for the suppliers, if individual managers telephone frequently and leave different names. The supplies officer should be the only person to whom the supplier relates.

The decision must be taken as to when each room is fully fitted out. I would suggest that this depends very much on the security available. It may be better to have all items delivered to a large, lockable room within the department, and only fit out each area during the last month prior to opening. As long as the lists are all checked off as the deliveries occur, problems should not arise. Consumable medical, surgical and pharmaceutical stock should be requisitioned to arrive two weeks before opening. Controlled drugs should not be brought into the department until it is occupied on a 24-hour basis. All stationery should be ordered and delivered two weeks prior to opening.

This timetable may seem a little tight to some. However, as long as the commissioning officer / head of department has worked closely with the supplies officer, then everything required within the department should be in stores well before the delivery date required.

1.6 PERSONNEL MANAGEMENT

Whether the department is an extension or refurbishment of an old one, a transfer from an older hospital, or a brand new department, personnel management is one of the most important parts of commissioning. Existing staff should be consulted and kept informed at all stages of the building and commissioning programme. Uncertainty and rumour undermine morale at the very time that extra effort and co-operation may be required from staff.

A move to a new building is a useful time to examine and review existing practice, and introduce those changes deemed desirable. There should be no change for change's sake; in fact, it may be better to only make one or two major changes until the running of the new department is determined.

With a totally new hospital, the advertising for staff will have to be planned according to the opening date. If the opening is delayed, staff may be in post for several weeks before the department is in use. This time should be put to good use. From the first day of opening, the staff will have to mould into a team and it is worthwhile allowing them time to get to know each other and the place they will be living in.

How many staff? This is always a difficult problem. The DHSS and Royal College of Nursing Accident and Emergency forum have looked at Accident Departments, and neither has come up with a recommendation for acceptable levels or gradings of staff. The yardstick to be used is that which provides a level for safe practice at all times. With the variation in workload of each Accident Department, no specific norms can be made. I believe that the permanent staff should all be trained. There is no good reason for having a Department overloaded with Sisters. Staff nurses should be undergoing development and training to take charge of a Department. The team situation allows for the further development of the enrolled nurse.

It must also be remembered when deciding on staff numbers that all Accident and Emergency Departments are experiencing a 5–10% increase in attendance rate annually and plans should make allowance for this. All experienced A and E staff will realize the bedevilment of 'new attendances'. These are the figures taken to look at workload. This author has long argued that total attendances, that is all figures, should be used to calculate staffing needs. After all, if

10% of the total workload are re-attendances of one type or another, they still require nursing time. This, of course, should also apply to all other budgets — new attendance numbers provide false yardsticks and are to be avoided.

Once staff have been recruited, then planned induction programmes must be arranged. If staff are moving from one building to another, induction programmes should still be held which will include orientation to the new department, working out patient movement to the best advantage, and teaching sessions with all new equipment. This should include hands-on experience so that staff are familiar with where equipment is kept and how it works before the first day of operation. It is at this stage that the staff who are to run the department can be most involved by putting forward ideas regarding day-to-day operations. One word of warning: once a decision has been made on where a particular piece of equipment is kept or on a certain method of doing something, that decision should be held for at least one year. Continual changes lead to confusion. Every department needs time to settle and all major changes should be left for discussion and amendment until time allows a proper appraisal.

Staff orientation and training sessions within the department should, however, be considered as one part of the whole. It is too easy to be insular; each area or department will be considering its function and naturally looking to find the most effective and efficient method of operation.

In an organization as complex as a hospital, all areas have to interlink. Heads of departments will be holding their meetings and discussing how they relate to each other. Other staff should also be encouraged to meet and learn how other departments work. It should, however, be made clear that this is not a backdoor way to modify how other departments will relate to A and E. Any potential problems should be brought back to the department head for discussion. It may be something that had already been considered, and because it is important at this stage to create good relationships for future working, diplomacy and tact are paramount. This must be stressed to staff. At this stage of commissioning, everyone is working at 110% and it is all too easy for innocent remarks to be misinterpreted. Staff should be encouraged always to use their line manager for discussion.

The staff training and orientation period is the ideal time to set the standards that will be expected for the future. Attitudes are quickly acquired and hard to lose or change, so the opportunity should be taken to set out exactly what will be required and how it will be achieved.

1.7 PATIENT SERVICES

Apart from the obvious medical and nursing service to be provided, there are all those other services that happen and that nurses do not usually consider. They all, however, are part of an efficient, well-run department and the department heads involved will meet together to analyze these. Again, it is useful to consider ideas from other members of staff with regard to these services. As each department, the area it serves, and the particular type of service it offers is different, it is not proposed to provide exhaustive detail regarding these, but rather a check list. The following are areas for consideration:

- admission and transfers: registration, documentation, reappointments, discharge letters
- admission to intensive care or coronary care units
- signposting to all areas
- triage room or desk
- waiting areas, supervised children's area
- sub-waiting areas, clinics, plaster room, x-ray room
- refreshment area
- distressed relatives' room
- toilet areas
- treatment areas with a sub-waiting room
- patient movement
- ambulance or other transport services; hospital car service
- transfer to other hospitals; medical and surgical referrals
- clinic facility policy
- resuscitation procedures
- laboratory and pharmacy services
- monitoring of children
- chaplain on call provision, to include all religious and ethnic groups in the area
- health and safety provision; accidents to patients or relatives
- containment of and dealing with violence; security, fire and

evacuation procedures
- rules about smoking
- infectious patients, or those with special needs
- patients brought in dead; liaison with coroner and mortuary
- drug addiction treatment and referral
- homeless patients
- dental, pharmacy, special clinics; off-hours service
- care of patients' property
- noticeboards, video screening for health education and patient services
- patient information leaflets, e.g. information on care of plasters or head injury
- provision of interpreters; provision of leaflets in various languages
- interview room for psychiatric services, social workers or police
- information to police or press
- liaison with community: district nurses, health visitors, psychiatric nurses, social workers
- liaison with local authority
- maintenance of equipment
- obtaining patient aids
- stores ordering and delivery
- home help and meal services
- provision of public telephones and one for private use by distressed relatives
- linen provision, portering and clerical services
- local taxi and bus service

1.8 PROCEDURES AND POLICIES

One of the most exciting parts of setting up a new department is the drawing up of new policies and procedures. This is the opportunity everyone dreams of — the ability to introduce those changes you have always wanted, to get away from that 'we've always done it this way' syndrome. It must be remembered, however, that not everything that went before was impractical or useless. The best must be retained while the rest is modified. Procedures for the treatment of minor and major injuries must be worked out in conjunction with relevant medical staff. The extended role of the nurse will be considered along with these. It is important at this stage to have this totally clarified.

In today's climate, many authorities tend to contract the role of the A and E nurse, often to the detriment of patient care. Many routine diagnostic and emergency treatments have been removed into the realm of medical care (e.g. blood sugars and plastering), whilst nurses are being expected to fulfil other roles. Accident and Emergency Departments are about team work, not demarcation, and it is important to the future of the service that this is realized.

The extended role policy should reflect this and be formulated by those who know what nurses do and what they are trained for. In discussions of Accident and Emergency policies, it has been noted that the Major Incident policy is often uppermost in everyone's thoughts. In fact, especially in a brand new department, this should probably be the last policy to be considered. The department needs to be opened and functioning satisfactorily before it becomes designated. A year after opening is probably a more realistic time to consider becoming designated as a Major Incident Centre.

All policies for a new department will need to consider the functioning of other parts of the hospital. They should be simple and written in basic clear English that is easy to remember and should include those parts of the overall district policies that are relevant. This can be done by the addition of a reference section, as district policies in total tend to be rather long and involved. Some policies can be written using the patient services check list (section 1.7).

It should be remembered that with changes in the law regarding patients' records, patients will have the right of access to their notes and a policy will need to be formulated in the light of legislation being introduced.

1.8.1 'Dry runs'

Prior to opening of the department, 'dry runs' must be carried out. It is useful to time how long it takes to transfer a patient to the furthermost ward, as this is the minimum length of time a nurse will be absent from the department. Transfers to specialist areas should also be practised.

If the co-operation of the other services is sought, it is often possible to have a morning dry run session with all the staff in the department acting out their roles and volunteers acting as patients.

Ambulance services will usually co-operate in this, as they too need to know how the new department will work. The dry run should not be held weeks before opening, because the build-up to opening day will be lost. Rather, it should be just before opening when every detail has been thrashed out and a decision has been taken that only very major faults will be amended. It is in the nature of things that people will find minor details that do not suit them, but someone has to say 'enough is enough' and so the decision is taken. As stated previously, the department should then be left to run for a year before evaluation.

1.8.2 Design in use

Part of the evaluation procedure of the department as a whole will be the design in use evaluation required by capital planners so that future projects can exclude those aspects found unsatisfactory. Defects found in structural items will come under the defects liability and the department head should make a list of these as they occur. It is not worthwhile calling the contractor for each small item. The commissioning team will still be in operation and the department head should liaise with them regarding defects.

Distinctions must be made between defects, for instance, taps not working, and those items the user now deems desirable, such as shelving. There is a moratorium on alterations, which may be six or twelve months, that will render the defect liability clause void if alterations are carried out. Many nurses will not be aware of this, and natural enthusiasm must be curbed until the moratorium period is over.

Evaluation of the design in use should be kept simple. It will look at the design lay-out and materials used to see how they have stood up to use and whether they should be included in any future designs. This is the time for nursing staff to look at their policies and procedures. One year after opening will reveal which need modification or improvement, or even discarding. This should be done in a planned way, not haphazardly and not all at once. Changes should evolve so that staff are not disrupted and are kept informed. Working parties can be set up so that staff can be involved in policy changes.

The Major Incident policy can also be considered at this time. A core group of nurses, medical staff and an administrator should draw up an outline and other groups can be co-opted as each area is considered. The police, fire and ambulance authorities should also be consulted as their plans must interlock with the hospital's. Adjacent hospitals that will serve as overflow or backup should also be consulted. A Major Incident plan should always be followed by a Major Incident practice so that problems can be ironed out. It is not, however, an appropriate time to re-vamp the whole plan. Major Incident plans should always be considered only as guidelines. No plan is foolproof and they all have one disadvantage: the victims and passers-by of a Major Incident have not read your plan, so the unexpected always happens.

Commissioning and bringing a new department to operation is exciting, frustrating, stimulating and exhausting. It is something many people will tackle only once in a career — many will say this is enough. It is, however, one of the most satisfying experiences to look back at a functioning department and know that your hard work helped to make it possible.

EDITOR'S NOTES

Despite a rigorous search I found little reference to nurses' input in the planning and commissioning of Emergency Departments. This chapter therefore is what innovation is all about — the excitement, the pitfalls and the sheer hard work are all here. It is desperately important that nurses are an integral part of this planning stage.

Although some provision is universal, local needs and the provision for them are also stressed here. It is for this reason I have suggested reading the document on health spending (O'Higgins) which concludes that provision for demographic fluctuations and major new illnesses such as AIDS should be accounted for. Jill Milnthorpe's comments about patients who leave without being seen in the Department after registration highlights the important need in certain areas for observation by nurses.

This chapter reminded me of other aspects of emergency care and their relation to each other: the need for a separate room for distresed relatives, for example, and for the management of violent patients. Careful planning results in effective management.

The managerial expertise of Emergency nurses and the need for training in this aspect of our work becomes evident when reading this chapter. Other issues are also highlighted, such as needing the ability to present our needs clearly and effectively to management. If we are to spend thousands of pounds we must be seen to have both knowledge and ability. I believe this chapter will help us to do this more effectively.

FURTHER READING

Körner (1982) *First Report* HMSO, London.
Miller, M.E. (1982) *Emergency Department Management.* C.V. Mosby, St. Louis.
O'Higgins, M. (1987) *Health Spending — A Way to Sustainable Growth.* RCN Publications, London.
Tortella, B.J. and Trunkey, D.D. (1984) Trauma care systems. *Trauma,* **1,** 1.
Weissberg, M.P., Hunter, M., Lowenstein, S. and Keefer, G. (1986) Patients who leave without being seen. *Annals of Emergency Medicine,* **15,** 1.
Yates, D.W. and Redmond, A.D. (1985) *Lecture Notes on Accident and Emergency Medicine.* Blackwell Scientific Publications, London.

2

Trauma Education for Nurses

Joseph Blansfield

2.1 OVERVIEW OF THE PROBLEM

Trauma, a word generally used to describe an injury or a wound, has become a problem that is reaching epidemic proportions in contemporary society. It is more costly both in terms of money and lives than any other disease that health care providers will treat. In order to gain a better appreciation of trauma as a 'neglected disease', I would like to compare and contrast some epidemiological aspects of trauma in the United States and in other countries.

The leading cause of death for Americans under the age of 40 is trauma. Overall, it is ranked third as a cause of death for all ages combined. It is only behind the more publicly recognized problems of heart disease and cancer, ranked first and second respectively. Trauma makes an impact not only on mortality figures but on morbidity figures as well. The data have shown that for each trauma death, there are two permanent disabilities. For example, there were 165,000 deaths and 325,000 permanent disabilities in 1982. In fact, combined trauma deaths (motor vehicle accidents, homicides and suicides) have risen by 50% since 1976 and there is no sign of letting up. The belief that the United States is a violent society is given further evidence by a death rate for teenagers and young adults that is 50% higher than for their contemporaries in Britain, Sweden, and Japan.[1]

Trauma can be accurately described as a young person's disease. Unfortunately it affects the age group of potentially productive contributors to society for many years to come. Trauma suddenly and catastrophically makes them dependents of that society.

Therefore, its costs can be measured in both the expense of health care for the trauma victim and his lost wages and services. This is estimated to be approximately $63 million per day in lost wages alone, or about $23 billion per year. Total costs including lost wages, medical expenses, and indirect losses such as property damage reach as high as $50 billion a year.[2]

Trauma presently accounts for about one-third of the 2 million hospital admissions in the United States each year. More patients are treated by Accident and Emergency personnel because of trauma than any other disease. At least one out of every five individuals will visit an Emergency Department during the year due to a trauma-related injury. Those patients who require admission will consume a total of 20 million hospital days each year, easily more than heart disease and four times more than cancer.[3]

2.2 STRATEGIES

It has been proposed that this problem should be addressed by three separate strategies: prevention, standardization and education. The first two are beyond the scope of this chapter and will be mentioned only briefly.

Prevention has been identified as the only way to reduce significantly the amount of morbidity and mortality that is associated with trauma. It is estimated that as many as 40% of all trauma deaths can be averted. This would require the introduction and popular support of various comprehensive prevention programmes, some of which may be seen as controversial. It is important to remember that public support is crucial for any trauma prevention campaign to be meaningful and effective. This task begins with increasing public awareness of the problem. I believe that nurses as health care professionals have an inherent role in patient teaching and public education. Nurses should consider themselves as trauma prevention advocates educating the public as to the magnitude of the problem and eliciting their support for trauma prevention. This is not an easy task. Several prevention programmes involve controversial social issues that may be perceived as an infringement upon personal liberties and therefore may not be readily embraced. The issues of drunk drivers, mandatory seat belts and helmets, handgun control and drug-related crimes are examples.

The issue of standardization involves the uniformity of trauma care delivery. During the 1970s the idea of designating certain hospitals and their Emergency Departments as 'trauma centres' began. The intent was to concentrate resources and personnel in one institution in order to effect a better outcome in trauma resuscitation. However, this meant that patients would no longer be brought to the nearest facility, but would go some extra distance to be brought to a more appropriate facility to provide more definitive care. After some reluctance due to political and fiscal reasons, the concept is now broadly established. Hospitals can be designated at different levels (I–IV) depending on their care capability.

There have also been successful attempts in standardizing injury assessments. Injuries can be categorized anatomically and physiologically according to their severity and complications. This allows the use of a uniform scale to determine which patients should be treated or transferred in order to provide for them the best care possible.

Trauma education is a very broad topic. It can take place at different levels and have different effects on learners depending on what their potential application of this knowledge will be. I would like to break this discussion into two parts. First, it is necessary to mention the various educational programmes in the United States available for nurses interested in practising trauma care. I will attempt to describe and give examples of each. Secondly, I will relate the experience of developing and implementing an educational programme focused specifically on the role of the nurse as part of a team resuscitation.

2.3 EDUCATIONAL PROGRAMMES

Trauma education as a specific academic topic for nurses exists at three levels. Space limitation does not allow a complete listing of nursing programmes currently available; therefore I can only provide a sampling of each.

2.3.1 Academic degrees at the graduate level[4]

This is currently the highest educational level specific to trauma nursing. It awards the Master of Science Degree in Nursing with a specialty in Trauma, Burn, Critical Care and/or Emergency Nursing. It is designed for those nurses who have completed a Bachelor of Science Degree programme and have obtained professional nursing experience within this specialty. Nurses who enroll in these programmes are usually those desiring expertise in trauma and emergency nursing. Career aspirations usually include clinical nurse specialists (expert clinicians), teachers, consultants and researchers, among others. Courses are offered at:

(a) University of Cincinnati College of Nursing and Health, Cincinnati, Ohio: Master of Science Degree in Medical-Surgical Nursing, with specialization in burn and trauma nursing
(b) University of Maryland, Baltimore, Maryland: Master of Science in Nursing in Trauma/Critical Care Nursing
(c) University of Texas Health Science Center, Houston, Texas: Master of Science in Nursing in Emergency Nursing
(d) University of Washington, Seattle, Washington: Master of Science in Nursing in Burn, Trauma and Emergency Nursing

2.3.2 Non-degree (trauma nurse specialist)[5]

These are concentrated clinically-oriented programmes presenting advanced concepts of trauma care. The complexities of initial assessments and the formulation of meaningful nursing interventions for the evaluation and treatment of the critically injured trauma patient are presented in detail. This type of programme is most useful for senior staff, head nurses and nurse educators seeking a broader understanding of trauma care and developing beginning teaching and nursing resource experience.

(a) Illinois Department of Public Health (nine sites in Illinois): Trauma Nurse Specialist Postgraduate Program, 4 weeks
(b) Parkway Regional Medical Center, North Miami Beach, Florida: Trauma Nurse Specialist Program, 4 weeks
(c) Maricopa Medical Center, Phoenix, Arizona: Emergency Trauma Nurse Specialist Program, 4 weeks
(d) Baystate Medical Center, Springfield, Massachusetts: Trauma Nurse Specialist Program, 8 weeks

2.3.3 Continuing education offerings (trauma course)

This type of programme is developed for the clinical nurse currently practising in an emergency setting who desires a concise and comprehensive programme that presents current information about trauma care delivery. The programme is usually fast-paced because of the time limitation. Therefore, the focus is on the most relevant and applicable content that may be brought back to the practice arena immediately. These nurses are seeking the knowledge and skills necessary to care effectively for the trauma victim and work with physicians to decrease trauma morbidity and mortality. I feel this group has the greatest opportunity to make a difference. Courses are offered at:

(a) Boston City Hospital, Boston, Massachusetts: Trauma Course, 2 days
(b) Bronson Methodist Hospital, Kalamazoo, Michigan: Nurse as Part of Trauma Team, 2 days
(c) Rhode Island Hospital, Providence, Rhode Island: Trauma Course, 2 days
(d) Maryland Institute for Emergency Medical Services Systems, Baltimore, Maryland: Trauma Nursing Triad, 3 days

2.4 TRAUMA COURSE DEVELOPMENT

In this section I will describe selected teaching principles and methods that I discovered were essential in the planning and implementation of a clinically-oriented trauma course for nurses. I will also detail the actual course objectives and content with their appropriate rationale and provide evaluation data from the courses presented thus far.

There are a few necessary considerations to keep in mind when planning an educational programme on trauma care. These notions were somewhat anticipated and eventually confirmed by the course presentation itself. First of all, it is fundamental that the teacher should have the ability to understand the material fully and be able to relate it to the participants at a level that they too can understand. Nurses want to come away from the programme with relevant and useful information that they can apply to their practice setting right away. Secondly, the faculty need to be able to speak from their own professional experience in order to establish credibility in both lecture and clinical skills. Illustrating a point by giving an example (case study) in which the speaker was personally involved generates more interest and comprehension. Previous teaching experience is certainly very helpful, but I believe that actual clinical experience is essential.

Lastly, it is necessary that the teacher generates a certain degree of enthusiasm for the material. The speaker must be convincing in her presentation, conveying the belief that an organized and enlightened approach to care of the trauma patient can make a difference. This course material and the manner in which it is presented can improve the nurses' clinical capability in trauma care and therefore their patients' outcomes.

2.4.1 Principles of adult learning

At this point, it will be helpful to review and discuss some of the principles of adult learning in order to help the adult educator to be optimally effective. Adult learning is largely the responsibility of the adult, who must find that the programme is helpful. The learner must actually perceive the need himself, because learning largely depends on motivation. Faculty can be most effective when acting as facilitators, creating the proper environment for the learning to take place.

The learning experience itself must be meaningful and relevant. The material should be directed at the learner's level of performance, allowing it to be perceived as practical and useful and encouraging greater application. It is helpful if the learner can describe real problems that have been encountered, so that the teacher and learner can work together finding meanings and resolutions.

Active involvement of the learner is essential. The level of interest of passive, nonparticipative adults will rapidly dwindle, and the attention spans may actually be shorter than those of children in some situations. Incorporating the application of knowledge into skills in teaching and testing situations maintains interest and increases involvement.

Succcessful learning requires ongoing feedback. Continuous evaluation of progress in both directions is very important for both learner and teacher. Feedback to the learner can be used to further improve and motivate performance while the teacher uses feedback to revise and refine teaching content and methods.[6]

2.4.2 Teaching methods

The teaching of a clinically oriented trauma course incorporating a number of skills requires several teaching methods in order to be effective. I will discuss those that were found to be most applicable.
Lecture is best used:

- simply to pass along information. This technique should not be used for reading; if the desire is for the learner to read something, give him a handout.
- to organize content in a specific way for a particular application, such as emergency nurses caring for a trauma patient 1–2 hours post-injury.
- to stimulate and develop learner interest in a subject. The learner's appreciation of the value of the material is vital to learning.
- to introduce content that will be developed and applied at a later time. This provides the theoretical foundation necessary to apply knowledge to skills.

Discussion is best used:

- to accomplish higher level objectives involving analysis, synthesis, and application of the material presented.
- to enlighten or alter the learner's attitudes, values or behaviours. These are slow to change and learners need to question, challenge and react in order to assimilate new learning.

Demonstration is best used:

- to teach psychomotor skills. Learners need to become familiar and comfortable with skills (especially those involving equipment) to perform effectively.
- to facilitate participation and group learning. Group involvement creates a social atmosphere that reduces stress and anxiety, and increases confidence.[7]

Audio visual aids are best used:

- to increase the amount of learning. Learners remember 10% of what they hear and 20% of what they see.

2.5 BOSTON CITY HOSPITAL TRAUMA COURSE

Boston City Hospital is a 450-bed general hospital attending over 50 000 patients in its Emergency Department each year. It is one of three designated trauma centres in the city of Boston, which means that the hospital receives the most seriously injured patients in its area. Approximately 1500 trauma patients are admitted each year. Two fully equipped trauma rooms are kept constantly ready to treat seriously ill and injured patients. Each day, members of the nursing and medical staffs are assigned to the Arrest Team. Members of the Arrest Team have predesignated roles and responsibilities which they fulfil whenever the team is called to the Trauma Room to treat patients admitted in Emergency.

The nursing staff in the Emergency Department have long been supportive of an organized team approach to trauma care. They have continued to organize and co-ordinate daily team meetings in which roles are reviewed and case management is discussed. Nursing considers this essential to provide consistency and quality care in the presence of a constantly changing resident physician staff.

At this time there is no standardized educational programme for Emergency nurses in trauma care. From the current literature and the collective experience of the clinical nursing staff we have learned that the effective method for the treatment of trauma patients is to prepare well co-ordinated staff to perform a series of preplanned assessment and management techniques.

The Boston City Hospital Trauma Course is a two-day educational programme providing Emergency nurses with the knowledge base and skill level to practise a standardized and systematic approach to the care of the trauma patient.

The course includes didactic and practice station components and competency testing. A course curriculum is comprised of lecture objectives, content outlines and bibliographies as well as evaluation and testing criteria. In order to enhance the educational presentation, a slide library was developed to correspond to and illustrate the lecture material. A variety of trauma equipment was acquired for the teaching and testing stations.

Faculty for the course are composed of members of the Boston City Hospital ED nursing staff. Lecturers are chosen for their emergency nursing expertise, teaching ability and willingness to participate in implementation of the course curriculum. The audience for the course is currently practising emergency nurses throughout the state of Massachusetts, with class size limited to 20 participants.

The course material presented on the first day is organized in a systems approach (see Appendix). Lectures are presented with an emphasis on material that is practical and can be readily applied to the clinical setting. In the afternoon, selected skills and equipment used in trauma care are demonstrated with practice time for the participants. In the skill stations, faculty explain that nurses and physicians share the same knowledge base in trauma care but apply it in a different perspective. For example, we do not teach nurses to perform thoracotomies, but we do instruct them to anticipate when a patient may need one, identify anatomical landmarks, utilize the appropriate equipment and monitor the patient's response to treatment.

The second day builds on the knowledge and skills presented in the first. It also includes content that may be considered novel for a trauma course such as this. We have introduced material on trauma epidemiology and prevention and on psychological aspects of trauma that have been well received. The Mega-Trauma station requires the nurse to function in a simulated trauma scenario as a team leader. This nurse must integrate cognitive knowledge and psychomotor skills to identify injuries, establish priorities, delegate responsibilities and initiate treatment. There is also a short post-course test.

Participant evaluation of the trauma course has been very favourable. Demand has exceeded supply and we routinely receive twice the number of applications for the course that we can accommodate. We have carefully reviewed all the evaluations and have made some course revisions based on them. Future plans for this project include videotaping actual team resuscitations of trauma patients for teaching purposes, and the development of an Instructor Course for selected nurses who have completed the programme and would be interested in expanding the number of courses presented to nurses in other areas.

EDITOR'S NOTES

The all-embracing aspect of work in the Emergency Department poses many problems when considering curriculum content. This insight into US educational programmes is relevant to all areas of the world where trauma education is an issue. Structures and methods are discussed usefully, whilst the fact that some countries and even areas within countries have clear individual needs is stressed. The chapter outlines various principles and systems, but emphasizes that in adult education the responsibility then lies with the nurse to seek knowledge of these sections. I believe this promotes motivation and the ability to look critically at the work of others.

In order to avoid separating practice from education too distinctly, I have included in the Further Reading details of trauma scoring. Of course, this is also linked closely with triage and pre-hospital care, and is vital to our trauma education.

APPENDIX: BOSTON CITY HOSPITAL TRAUMA COURSE PROGRAMME SCHEDULE

Day one
8:00–8:15	Registration/Pre-Course Test
8:15–8:30	Opening remarks and course overview
8:30–9:30	Initial Assessment
9:30–10:30	Head and Central Nervous System Trauma
10:30–11:00	Break
11:00–12:00	Chest Trauma
12:00–1:00	Abdominal, Renal and Obstetric Trauma
1:00–2:00	Lunch
2:00–3:00	Musculoskeletal Trauma
3:00–5:00	Teaching Stations

Assessment and Resuscitation
　　Primary and secondary survey, Cervical spine immobilization
　　Airway management, Chest decompression
Stablization and Management
　　Helmet removal, Central venous pressure lines, Pericardiocentesis
　　Peritoneal lavage, Splints, PASG (pneumatic anti-shock garment)

Day two
8:00–9:00	Trauma Physiology
9:00–10:00	Trauma Epidemiology and Prevention
10:00–10:15	Break
10:15–11:00	Pediatric Trauma
11:00–11:45	Psychotrauma
11:45–12:30	Team Resuscitation/Patient Transport
12:30–1:30	Lunch

1:30–4:30   Testing Stations
Mega-Trauma
Mega-Trauma is composed of five testing stations. The nurse is to apply knowledge and skills of nursing assessment and management in simulated trauma situations. Each nurse will function as a team leader, identifying injuries, establishing priorities, delegating responsibilities and demonstrating selected techniques using trauma resuscitation equipment. Examples of the five stations may include a:

1. motorcyle accident with head and severe extremity injuries;
2. thirty-foot fall with pelvic fracture, abdominal and genito-urinary trauma;
3. gunshot wound to right chest with respiratory distress and deviated trachea;
4. motor vehicle accident with chest contusions and femur fracture; and
5. multiple stab wounds to left chest and neck with dyspnea and expanding hematoma.

Each nurse will proceed through three randomly selected stations: one for practice, one for critique, and one for testing. Time is also allotted for demonstrations, skills practice and a written post-course test. Course evaluations are completed at the end of the programme.

REFERENCES

1. Trunkey, D.D. (1983) 'Trauma'. *Scientific American*, **249**, 28–35.
2. Ibid.
3. Ibid.
4. Trunkey, D.D. (1985) 'Emergency nursing education programs'. *Journal of Emergency Nursing*, **11**, 20A–22A.
5. Ibid.
6. Committee on Trauma, American College of Surgeons (1984) *Advanced Trauma Life Support Course Instructor Manual*, American College of Surgeons, Chicago, Illinois.
7. Ibid.

FURTHER READING

Cales, R.H. (1985) Trauma scoring and prehospital triage. *Annals of Emergency Medicine*, **14**, 11.

Ferguson, D.C. and Lord, S.M. (1986) *Practical Procedures in Accident and Emergency Medicine*. Butterworth, London.

Ferrer, J. (1987) Developing post-basic clinical nursing courses. *Care of the Critically Ill*, **3**, 1.

Kilne, G. *et al*. (1986) Comparison of a videotape instructional programme with traditional lectures for medical student emergency medical training. *Annals of Emergency Medicine*, **15**, 1.

Smith, L. (1982) Models of nursing as the basis for curriculum development: some rationale and implication. *Journal of Advanced Nursing*, **7**, 117–27.

Steedman, D. and Robertson, C. (1987) Who scores in trauma. *Care of the Critically Ill*, **3**, 3.

3

Professional Development of Nursing Practice

Dianne M. Danis

3.1 INTRODUCTION

The professional development of emergency nursing is occurring rapidly. This chapter attempts to explain how that development is advanced and applied where it really matters — in the Emergency Department (ED). In order for patients to benefit, theories and trends must be translated into nursing care systems and programmes. The person who can make this happen is the ED nurse manager, whether called nurse manager, head nurse, chief nurse, or assistant director of nursing. The role of the nurse manager reflects the synthesis of conceptualization and implementation.

The first section of this chapter, The Practice of Emergency Nursing, provides an overview of the current status of emergency nursing. The second section, The Management of Emergency Nursing, describes how to manage so that an emphasis can be placed on excellence in emergency nursing. The last section, Professional Development in the ED, discusses several of the nursing programs in progress at the Boston City Hospital (BCH) ED. These programmes are an example of one ED's attempt to transform concepts into practice.

3.2 THE PRACTICE OF EMERGENCY NURSING

Over the last 15 years, emergency nursing in the United States has become recognized as a nursing specialty, with a unique body of knowledge and skills. Today, the specialty is still evolving.

However, the practitioners of today have clearly described standards of excellence towards which to strive.

Emergency nursing is grounded in the general precepts of nursing. 'Nursing is the diagnosis and treatment of human responses to actual or potential health problems,' according to the American Nurses Association (1980:9). These human responses may include self-care limitations, impaired bodily functioning, pain, emotional problems, self-image changes and stresses related to life processes. Nursing practice is actualized through a problem-solving approach known as the nursing process, which involves assessment, diagnosis, planning, intervention and evaluation.

The definition of emergency nursing practice in the US is an elaboration of the definition of nursing promulgated by the American Nurses Association. Emergency nursing practice is 'the assessment, diagnosis and treatment of human responses to perceived, actual or potential, physical or psychosocial problems that may be episodic, primary and/or acute' (Emergency Department Nurses Association [ENA] 1983:3). It is obvious that the emergency nurse must be skilled in a broad range of interventions. For example, Thompson (1984) describes several types of emergency nursing activities in which the emergency nurse should possess or develop expertise:

- physiological care of emergency (critically ill or injured) patients
- psychological and supportive care of emergency patients and their families
- physiological assessment, intervention and continual monitoring for non-emergency patients
- support, reassurance and education to non-emergency patients
- reassurance and education for families of non-emergency patients
- education, support and referral for 'repeaters' (patients who repeatedly return for treatment)
- patient education concerning self-assessment, self-care and community resources
- public education concerning injury prevention, first aid and use of emergency facilities

The development of emergency nursing in the US has been spearheaded by the specialty nursing association (ENA) founded in 1970. ENA publishes the *Journal of Emergency Nursing*, a bi-monthly publication. It conducts an annual national educational meeting with three days of clinical and professional programmes. It has developed a core curriculum (ENA, 1980–85) for emergency nursing that provides learning modules — behavioural objectives, content outlines, teaching strategies and evaluation methods — for every area of emergency nursing. It sponsors a competency-based certification examination, the successful completion of which allows the nurse to use the designation CEN (Certified Emergency Nurse). Perhaps most important, ENA has published the *Standards of Emergency Nursing Practice* (1983).

3.2.1 Standards of Emergency Nursing Practice

The ENA *Standards*, published in 1983, were a significant development. They define the criteria that exemplify excellence in practice. According to the *Standards*, emergency nursing involves the integration of four essential concepts: practice, research, education and professionalism. Each is operationalized in the *Standards* by one or more comprehensive standards, displayed in Table 3.1. Comprehensive standards are further defined by rationale and outcome and by specific component standards and outcome criteria. For example, Table 3.2 contains the entire standard for administration.

The first of the four concepts — practice — has been defined above. Its eight comprehensive standards contain numerous statements that delineate the nature of modern emergency nursing. For example, they recommend:

- triage of all patients
- formulation of nursing diagnoses
- development of standardized care plans
- conduct of case reviews
- use of standardized teaching plans and written aftercare instructions
- development of a quality assurance plan
- conduct of patient care conferences for repeater patients

Research is defined as the 'discovery and verification of knowledge on which the practice of the specialty is based' (ENA 1983:3). According to the research standard, emergency nurses should use information from the research literature to improve their practice, should conduct and support research, and should conform to the ethical standards governing research.

Table 3.1 Comprehensive standards of ENA *Standards of Emergency Nursing Practice*

PRACTICE STANDARDS

Knowledge and Skills: Emergency nurses shall possess current comprehensive knowledge and skills.

Assessment: Emergency nurses shall initiate accurate and ongoing assessment of physical and psychosocial problems of patients.

Analysis: Emergency nurses shall analyze assessment data to formulate a nursing diagnosis.

Planning: Emergency nurses shall formulate a comprehensive nursing care plan and collaborate in the formulation of the overall patient care plan.

Intervention: Emergency nurses shall implement a plan of care based on assessment data as well as a sound knowledge base.

Evaluation: Emergency nurses shall evaluate and modify the plan of care based on observable responses of patients and attainment of patient goals.

Human Worth: Emergency nurses shall provide care based on philosophical and ethical concepts and on a resolution to act dynamically in relation to people's beliefs.

Communication: Emergency nurses shall assure open and timely communication with emergency patients, their significant others, and team members.

RESEARCH STANDARDS

Emergency nurses shall recognize and value research as a methodology to further emergency nursing practice.

EDUCATION STANDARDS

Provision of Information: Emergency nurses shall assist the patient and significant others to obtain knowledge about illness and injury prevention and treatment.

Education of Self and Peers: Emergency nurses shall recognize their own learning needs and those of their peers and assist in meeting those needs to maximize professional development and optimal emergency nursing practice.

PROFESSIONALISM STANDARDS

Qualifications: Emergency nurses shall be competent and current, adhering to established standards of practice.

Professional Status: Emergency nurses shall engage in a variety of activities and behaviours that characterize professionals.

Administration: Emergency nurses in management shall function in collegial relationships with other administrators having responsibilities in the emergency care setting.

Communication: Emergency nurses shall actively communicate with team members in the emergency care system.

Source: Standards of Emergency Nursing Practice (ENA 1983).

Table 3.2 Professionalism Standard III: Administration

Standard III: Emergency nurses in management shall function in collegial relationships with other administrators having responsibilities in the emergency care setting.

Rationale: Inherent in the delivery of emergency care is the phenomenon of collegial and collaborative participation by varied health care professionals. Hence it is essential that policy decisions and communications at the management level are both collegial and reciprocal.

Outcome: Emergency nurses in management:

- are the ultimate decision makers on issues regarding emergency nursing
- are recognized as peers by other managers with responsibilities in the emergency care setting
- direct, develop and implement policies, procedures and standards governing emergency nursing practice

Components Standards	*Outcome Criteria*
A. Job description: Emergency nurses shall have a job description that reflects current standards of professional practice and lists specific responsibilities	A. 1 Job descriptions are available at the time of interview. 2 Job descriptions are utilized in performance review. 3 Emergency nurses have input into periodic revision of job descriptions.
B Performance review: Emergency nurses' performance shall be reviewed by emergency nurses in management, based on identified roles and responsibilities.	B. 1 The review contains input from the individual being reviewed and other appropriate health professionals. 2 Emergency nurses are evaluated on a periodic basis. 3 Emergency nurses' modification of practice in accordance with performance appraisal is reviewed.

C Staffing: Emergency nurses in management shall take measures to ensure provision of adequate staffing of qualified professional nurses to provide for safe care.

C. 1 The level of staffing reflects recognition of variables that affect the delivery of safe, effective emergency nursing care.

2 Staffing patterns are reviewed regularly by emergency nurses in management to ensure delivery of safe, effective emergency care.

3 Staffing patterns provide adequate time for:

- triage, assessment, intervention, and evaluation of intervention
- crisis intervention
- patient and significant others referral and aftercare instructions
- breaks and mealtimes

Source: Standards of Emergency Nursing Practice (ENA, 1983) pp. 61–2.

The third component — education — involves ongoing education of oneself and teaching of patients, families, the community and other members of the emergency care team. According to the *Standards*, patient teaching should be carried out concerning medications, treatments, self-care, referral and/or prevention; pertinent written instructions should also be provided.

The last component is professionalism. The characteristics of professionalism are defined as accountability, autonomy, authority and leadership. The four comprehensive standards recommend:

- a Baccalaureate degree in nursing (ideally)
- twelve hours of continuing education annually
- certification in emergency nursing within two years of employment
- a written job description
- performance reviews incorporating self-evaluation and peer evaluation
- regular review of staffing patterns for adequacy

The ENA *Standards* provide a blueprint for emergency nursing practice. They allow evaluation of current practice and planning for the future.

3.3 THE MANAGEMENT OF EMERGENCY NURSING

Nurses who are responsible for ED nursing services have a difficult task. The nurse manager is expected to keep the department running smoothly, keep costs in line, provide adequate staffing, satisfy regulatory requirements, prevent and/or solve problems and ensure the delivery of quality nursing care. In addition to the fact that these roles and responsibilities are numerous and sometimes conflicting, the nurse manager must function in an ED environment that is crisis-ridden, constantly changing and often chaotic. Nurse managers frequently find their time is occupied with 'putting out fires': problem management and crisis intervention. It is difficult to focus on long-range plans, implementing change, or programme development. This situation is frustrating for the nurse manager who wants to foster professional development and improve the practice of emergency nursing.

One solution to this dilemma is to adopt a managerial aproach called management by objectives (MBO). The remainder of this section describes MBO, outlines the MBO process and presents the application of MBO in an ED setting.

3.3.1 What is MBO?

MBO is a management strategy defined by Bell as a 'system for setting organizational objectives for a given period, devising plans to meet the objectives, and providing periodic evaluation of progress' (1980:19). MBO fosters achievement and progress, rather than the status quo. The concept is very simple, but it works.

MBO has many possible uses. They include:

- structuring a logical, comprehensive management system
- emphasizing both short- and long-range planning
- producing a pro-active, results-oriented approach
- preventing crisis-focused management
- fostering priority-setting and work planning

- increasing productivity and supplying an antidote to procrastination
- encouraging teamwork and a participative management style
- improving task delegation
- defining a format for supervising and developing subordinates
- providing criteria for performance subordinates

Many of the uses of MBO translate into advantages for the ED nurse manager. The programme emphasizes thoughtful planning, realistic objectives and goal achievement. All of these attributes will help to counteract the devotion of all one's time and energy to crisis management and problem-solving.

3.3.2 The MBO process

There are many variations of MBO (Bell 1980; Deegan and O'Donovan 1982; Drucker 1954; Pollok 1983). One of the advantages of the system is that it may be adapted to any setting for use by entire institutions, individual departments or individual managers. Once familiar with the concept, managers are encouraged to create a version of MBO that will work for them.

Generally, the MBO process starts with assessment and analysis. In the ED, the current status of the department should be assessed and external standards analyzed. During assessment, the following factors should be considered: patient population, level of nursing practice, budget, staffing, efficiency and productivity, environment, resources, support services, intra- and interdepartmental relationships and quality assurance. The manager should then analyse how well the department conforms to external standards for licensing or recognition. In addition to the ENA *Standards*, other standards applicable to the ED setting should be reviewed (American College of Emergency Physicians 1982–83; Joint Commission on Accreditation of Hospitals 1984).

After assessment and analysis, goals for the department should be established. Goals are general statements with a long-range perspective. They often describe improvements to be made, changes to be implemented and new roles or programmes to be developed. In essence, they describe the way a department should be or will be.

Once a list of general goals has been developed, objectives and action plans should be written. Objectives specify activities designed to further achievement of a goal. Each goal may have none, one or more than one related objective. Objectives should be specific, measurable, time-limited and, above all, *realistic*. Their subject matter may be routine, problem-solving, innovative or personal. Some objectives may benefit from the development of associated action plans. An action plan is a procedure for accomplishing an objective that includes the person responsible, the steps to be taken and target dates.

Operationalization and evaluation are the most important steps in the MBO process because it is here that plans are transformed into achievements. In many organizations these steps never take place and goals remain abstract concepts, written but never implemented.

The nurse manager can avoid this outcome by a commitment to set realistic goals, have patience with the process, recognize achievements, continually focus attention on the goals and conduct regular progress reviews. Goals and objectives can be discussed at management, supervisory and staff meetings, performance evaluations and in annual reports. Goals and objectives should be reviewed annually, their achievement evaluated, and they should be updated for the coming year.

3.3.3 Application of MBO in one ED

MBO has been used by the author in the ED at BCH since 1982. Familiarly referred to as the 'G and Os' (goals and objectives), MBO has provided us with structure, direction, control, progress and continuity. The G and Os have helped us to focus on life beyond the immediate crisis and to be more productive whenever we do have time between crises.

Our process is quite simple. We have a list of general goals (see Table 3.3), which are reviewed annually and revised when indicated. During the annual review, both ongoing programmes and new activities are discussed. Each member of the nursing leadership team takes responsibility for a few goals. Sometimes staff nurses will also have goals. The person responsible then develops more specific objectives (or action plans) for their assigned goals. As an example, Table 3.4 displays the objectives developed for the management goal.

Attention is focused on the G and Os by making them an agenda item during monthly group management meetings and individual supervision sessions. Progress is reviewed during performance

Table 3.3 Emergency department nursing goals, 1985–86.

1. To ensure the delivery of quality nursing care through such mechanisms as the:

   Standardized Care Plan Committee
   Policy/Procedure Committee
   Quality Assurance Committee
   Discharge Planning and Patient Teaching Task Force
   Certification/recertification
   Patient follow-up programme
   Case review and patient care conferences

2. To facilitate the continuing professional development of the staff through such mechanisms as the:

   Orientation programme
   Continuing education programme
   Performance evaluation system
   Recognition of excellence in nursing

3. To expand and refine the nursing management systems in the Emergency Department

4. To participate in and contribute to the larger organizational structures within the Department of Health and Hospitals

5. To enhance the reputation of the nursing staff by contributing to the professional nursing community and the lay community

Source: Compiled by the author.

evaluations and the annual report. The leadership team knows that the assistant director of nursing is committed to the goals and their achievement.

Achievement is emphasized, but support and encouragement are also necessary. During busy weeks in the department, there may be no time to devote to goal achievement. At best, several hours a month may be available. For this reason, it is important that the number of goals is limited, and that objectives are written in achievable increments. Any achievement, no matter how small, deserves recognition and applause.

At the end of each year, progress is evaluated preparatory to

Table 3.4 Objectives for Goal III, nursing management systems.

Goal III: To expand and refine the nursing management systems in the Emergency Department.

Objectives:

1. By September, to complete development of staffing/scheduling guidelines and delegation to head nurses responsible for this function

2. By September, to complete preparations for accreditation survey

3. By September, to compile a library of management articles for head nurses

4. By November, to organize an orderly transition for the co-ordinator's leave

5. By January, to develop guidelines for follow-up of incidents and complaints to achieve a more organized system

6. By April, to develop and implement a Charge Nurse Leadership Course

7. On an ongoing basis, to analyze and enhance the relationships between the adult and paediatric Emergency Departments

8. On an ongoing basis, to participate in the interhospital Patient Classification Task Force

Source: Compiled by the author.

writing the annual report and next year's goals. Looking back, our aims have often been somewhat ambitious and our progress slower than we would have liked, but over time our achievements have been steady. Each of the leadership team can take pride in contributing to excellence in emergency nursing.

3.4 PROFESSIONAL DEVELOPMENT IN THE ED

After identification of standards and trends, and establishment of goals and objectives, an individualized professional development programme will emerge. This section describes some of the professional development activities undertaken in the ED at BCH.

The activities are intended to foster excellence in nursing practice in the department. The total programme, as reflected in its goals and objectives (Table 3.3), is multifaceted. It emanates from modern standards and trends, regulatory requirements and the unique environment of the ED and the hospital.

The BCH ED is a busy, often hectic, department. The hospital is a city teaching hospital and the patients are predominantly of lower socioeconomic status. The hospital is a Trauma Center and the ED treats a great number of trauma patients, primarily the victims of interpersonal violence. Although municipal finances and resources are often limited, the nursing staff are competent and committed.

This section will discuss the goals and activities related to standardized care plans, quality assurance, patient follow-up, patient care conferences, continuing education, recognition of excellence and patient classification. Each goal will be discussed from both a general and a specific perspective. The general perspective will provide an overview of current thinking on a topic, while the specific perspective will describe the activity as it is implemented in the BCH ED.

3.4.1 Standardized Care Plans

(a) *Overview*

A standardized care plan (SCP) is 'a plan of care development for patients with a specific chief complaint' (ENA 1983:6). SCPs serve as general references to guide nursing care for certain types of patients, such as those with asthma or seizures. SCPs are an outgrowth of the planning component of the nursing process. First used for hospitalized patients, they have more recently been developed for the ED setting (Heister, Johnson and Trimberger 1982). According to the ENA *Standards*, 'emergency nurses shall develop and utilize standardized care plans as a systematic, uniform, and consistent method to provide safe and effective patient care' (1983:21). The *Journal of Emergency Nursing* recently initiated a helpful series of articles describing SCPs developed by different EDs (Neff 1985).

SCPs have many uses. They are labour-saving devices because the nurse does not have to create a new plan for each patient. They produce greater consistency because the entire staff is oriented to the same standard, and better quality because study, thought and debate are devoted to each topic. They are teaching tools that can be used to orientate new staff. They facilitate quality assurance and provide criteria for audits. However, it is important to recognize that patients may have additional individual requirements for nursing care.

Table 3.5 Standardized care plan for cardiac chest pain: excerpts from Assessment and disposition sections.

Assessment	Diagnosis	Plan/Intervention	Evaluation
Triage Assessment			
A. *One-second once-over for classic symptoms of myocardial infarction:* Severe, crushing midsternal chest pain Diaphoresis Pallor, cyanosis, ashen colour Decreased level of consciousness Severe shortness of breath Weak, thready pulse	A. *Probable cardiac event*	A. Trauma room or acute side	A. Document significant assessment findings
B. Assess for cardiac chest pain Symptom assessment[1]: Quality: crushing heaviness in chest 'gas-like' feeling Location: midsternal epigastric left-sided; difficult to localize left shoulder/arm	B. *Probable cardiac event* High probability: 5 or more symptoms Low probability: 4 or fewer symptoms	Acute side Nonacute side: obtain cardiogram and physician expeditiously	
Physical assessment Pulse: quality, rate, regularity Blood pressure in both arms Respirations: rate, difficulty Auscultate lungs for fluid			

Radiation:
  left arm
  left jaw
  back
Duration:
  several minutes to hours
  intermittent or constant
Precipitant:
  stress
  activity
  none
Associated signs/symptoms:
  shortness of breath
  nausea/vomiting
  pallor
  dizziness/syncope/lightheadedness
Pain not alleviated by:
  nitroglycerine
  rest
Risk factors:
  cardiac history
  age/sex
  sedentary life
  family history
  smoker
  drug abuse
  hypertension, diabetes

Table 3.5 (cont'd)

Assessment	Diagnosis	Plan/Intervention	Evaluation
C. *Assess for pleuritic chest pain* Symptom assessment[1]: pain with inspiration shortness of breath recent respiratory infection productive cough, thick yellow/brown/green sputum Physical assessment: auscultate breath sounds bilaterally for asymmetry, fluid, wheezes assess respiratory rate and effort	C. *Probable respiratory event* (pneumonia, pulmonary embolus, pneumothorax, pericarditis)	C. Acute side Immediate physician evaluation Chest x-ray as ordered	
D. *Assess for musculoskeletal pain* Symptom assessment[1]: pain easily localized duration (days to years) increase with movement Physical assessment: palpate for local tenderness	*Probable musculoskeletal event*	Nonacute side	
Disposition			
Discharged patient Assess patient/family knowledge: condition treatment regimen cardiac risk factors	Knowledge deficit	Identify learner readiness Initiate teaching: treatment and medica-	Document teaching and understanding of teaching

Assessment	Nursing diagnosis	Interventions	Documentation
Assess compliance: medication and treatment lifestyle changes activity follow-up cardiac risk factors	Noncompliance	Discuss cause: knowledge deficit financial need other Reinforce rationale for compliance with patient/family Refer to primary care provider	Document compliance status and follow-up
Assess patient/family anxiety and coping	Anxiety or coping deficit	Provide emotional support to family/patient Use psychiatric nurse as resource Use teaching to reduce anxiety Refer to support services for additional resources	Document emotional status and interventions

Table 3.5 (cont'd)

Assessment	Diagnosis	Plan/Intervention	Evaluation
Assess need for support services	Health care management deficit	Arrange appropriate support services: Veteran Nurses Association transportation home home health care lifeline MedicAlert bracelet referral to cardiac clinical nurse specialist	Document support service referrals

Source: Boston City Hospital *Standardized Care Plan for Chest Pain.*

[1]If the Symptom Assessment is positive, proceed with Physical Assessment. If the Symptom Assessment is negative, proceed with next Symptom Assessment.

(b) *Implementation*

Several SCPs have been developed at BCH since the formation of a committee for this purpose in 1983. The committee is composed of clinical nurses but is chaired by the clinical nurse specialist.

The care plans identify both medical and nursing diagnoses, and define assessment, intervention and evaluation in an emergency nursing process format. SCPs have been completed on nursing care of the patient with asthma, the patient with seizures or head injury, the pregnant patient with vaginal bleeding and the patient with cardiac chest pain. A plan for the intoxicated patient is currently being developed.

The topics of the care plans are common patient problems identified by the committee. One committee member develops a draft of each plan and then the entire committee reviews and refines the draft. The draft is also presented to the nursing staff and nursing management before a final version is adopted. Table 3.5 contains excerpts from the SCP for chest pain.

In 1985, the committee published an article on SCPs in the *Journal of Emergency Nursing* (Blansfield, Fackler and Bergeron) that described the process for SCP development.

3.4.2 Quality assurance

(a) *Overview*

Quality assurance (QA) refers to measures to assess and improve the quality of care. QA programmes have been strongly emphasized by the US Joint Commission on Accreditation of Hospitals (JCAH) as a requirement for hospital accreditation. Emergency and nursing services are both required by JCAH to have QA programmes. The ENA *Standards* also outlines components of emergency nursing QA programmes.

JCAH (1984) requires that the 'quality and appropriateness' of 'all major clinical functions' of care be assessed. Objective criteria are to be monitored on a routine basis; when problems are identified, problem-solving activities should be carried out, documented and evaluated.

The ENA *Standards* (1983) requires that each emergency nursing service develop a QA plan. The plan should be characterized by an organized approach to problem-solving. The following elements are suggested:

- review of patient complaints
- review of input from other health and community services agencies
- incident reports review
- multidisciplinary case reviews
- regular evaluation of care provided to repeaters

Specific emergency nursing QA studies and monthly chart audits are also discussed. In particular, audits should be conducted to validate SCPs.

As demonstrated by the literature, these general requirements have been fulfilled by a multitude of thoughtful, often creative approaches (Heister, Johnson and Trimberger 1982; Murphy and Jacobson 1984; Walts and Blair 1983).

(b) *Implementation*

The ED nursing QA committee is chaired by the clinical coordinator and consists of several members of the nursing staff. The committee has been involved in a number of episodic and ongoing QA activities. Three will be discussed here: SCP audits, return visit studies and an elopement study.

SCP Audits. As each SCP is developed, the SCP committee works with the QA committee to ensure that the criteria are clear, objective and measurable. After the care plan has been implemented, the QA committee conducts a chart audit. Charts are audited from time periods before and after introduction of the care plan. The results of each audit are compared and analyzed. These results are used to generate recommendations to nursing staff, the SCP committee and nursing management. At times, documentation (and presumably nursing care) has been shown to comply well with an SCP, while at other times gaps have been identified. Additional staff education might be needed, or perhaps some elements of the SCP need to be reconsidered.

Return Visit Study. The return visit study has uncovered some surprising results. It was felt that some patients, especially those with asthma and seizure disorders, were returning for care very frequently. The question arose as to whether they were receiving optimal nursing and medical care.

The committee wanted to analyze the characteristics of these repeater patients to see if we could improve our nursing care and decrease the frequency of these patients' visits. The first group studied were asthma patients and the results were quite surprising. All asthma patients seen in a one-month-period were noted and those who returned for a second visit within one week were identified. It turned out that very few patients returned within that time period, which seems to indicate that patients are receiving adequate care on their first visit. Out of 92 patients, only six returned within one week. Seizure patients were also analyzed with similar results: of 86 patients, only three returned. Since the results were much better than expected, it appears that nurses may have misconceptions about some repeater patients.

Elopement Study. The committee is currently conducting a study of patients who elope (leave) before their treatment is completed. Data are being gathered concerning number of elopements, time, department level of activity, chief complaint, waiting time and other variables. Although the study is not complete, it is apparent that the information gained will be very useful in addressing this problem.

3.4.3 Patient follow-up

(a) *Overview*

Patient satisfaction and continuity of care are two issues that have recently received a great deal of attention. Patient satisfaction has become a concern because of increasing competition for patients (for financial reasons), while improvements in continuity of care have been sought due to cost-containment pressures. EDs have begun to respond to both of these phenomena (Frank and McGovern 1983; Vestal 1984). In spite of the economic motivation for these trends, it is hoped that improved patient care will be the outcome.

One programme that fosters both patient satisfaction and continuity of care is a patient follow-up programme. Both JCAH (1984) and the ENA *Standards* (1983) require that patients be notified if it is discovered after discharge that they have abnormal laboratory studies, x-rays or electrocardiograms. In addition to these medical reasons, however, there are nursing reasons to follow up on ED patients. Anxious or intoxicated patients may be prone to forget instructions and complicated instructions may need reinforcement. There may be uncertainty as to whether patients are really able to return home, it may be particularly important for a patient to keep follow-up appointments, or the nurse may simply want to see how a patient is doing.

(b) *Implementation*

In 1985, BCH initiated a nursing telephone follow-up programme for ED patients. The programme is still in its initial phases but the phone calls have elicited positive responses from both nurses and patients.

The goal of the programme is to provide better follow-up and continuity of care for patients after they leave the ED. When the nurses are concerned about a patient they register her name in a logbook. Within the next day or two, one of the nurses will call the patient to see how she is doing and to encourage her to comply with aftercare instructions. We hope that, when fully implemented, this programme will result in improved patient care as well as a more positive public image for the department.

3.4.4 Patient care conferences

(a) *Overview*

Every ED has a group of repeaters, or frequent visitors. While some of these patients use the department appropriately, others do not. 'Inappropriate' patients — whether manipulative, noncompliant or disruptive — cause a great deal of frustration among ED staffs. In spite of their frequent visits, repeaters do not seem to improve.

The ENA *Standards* (1983:30) states that repeaters should be 'evaluated periodically to determine consistent and appropriate approaches and strategies'. One strategy for improving care of repeaters is to hold a patient care conference and develop a care plan (Cousins 1984; Rich 1982).

(b) *Implementation*

In our ED, the conference and care plan approach has been used for several patients, and in each instance this strategy has resulted in an improvement in the situation. In this process, nursing staff identify patients who need conferences. Usually these are patients with behavioural problems, although any frequent visitor with complex nursing and/or medical needs would benefit. The nurse manager or clinical nurse specialist then schedules a patient care conference.

The conferences are multidisciplinary. Participants include nurses, physicians, psychiatric nurses and social workers. The patient's medical record and pattern of ED visits are reviewed before the conference.

During the conference, information about the patient is shared and the patient's needs and problems discussed. Various strategies are identified to address these needs. Typically, each staff member has been trying a different approach with the patient, resulting in inconsistency and confusion. Often, the simple initiation of a standard approach to medical and nursing management eliminates confusion and sets clear limits for the patient. Primary nurses are also often identified to assume major responsibility for the patient and ensure that the standard approach will be achieved. In this way, nurses who choose to care for the patient take the burden off those who do not.

After the conference, a written care plan is completed and disseminated. A close watch is kept on subsequent patient visits to evaluate progress and reinforce the use of the care plan.

Each patient has responded to the conference and care plan approach. Some have improved their behaviour for varying periods of time while others have stopped coming to the ED. It is unknown whether they have simply chosen another ED. In all cases, patient management has been simplified, and staff frustration relieved.

3.4.5 Continuing education

(a) *Overview*

US emergency nurses merit a considerable investment in continuing education for two reasons. First, generic nursing education programmes contain little or no training in emergency nursing. Second, advances in emergency care require ongoing education in order for nurses to remain competent.

Sources of continuing education are many. Programmes are offered at the national, regional and state level, locally and at the hospital level. Sponsors include professional organizations, private companies, educational institutions, hospital consortia and individual hospitals. Seminars and short courses are the most common, with fewer long courses. With certain exceptions, there is little standardization from state to state regarding educational programming for emergency nurses.

(b) *Implementation*

A rather extensive educational programme has been designed for BCH ED nurses, to ensure that the staff possess the clinical concepts essential to competent practice. The programmes are coordinated by the clinical nurse specialist. Several standard programmes are supplemented by shorter conferences on various topics offered periodically. Standard programmes include orientation, preceptor and triage courses, the Critical-Care Emergency Department Nurse Education Programme (CEDNEP), and the BCH Trauma Nurse Course (TNC).

Orientation and Preceptorship. Orientation for new ED nurses is approximately two months in length. After two weeks of general hospital orientation and introduction to the unit, approximately six weeks are spent by the new nurse working with an experienced senior nurse who serves as preceptor. The orientation is tailored to the individual nurse's strengths and weaknesses and different nurses attain independence at different points during the six-week period. Although little formal teaching is conducted, a great deal of informal teaching occurs.

Senior nurses are provided with a four-hour educational programme, to help them become better preceptors. The programme contains information on principles of learning and teaching, leadership, communication skills and expectations of the preceptor role. Faculty include the clinical nurse specialist, nurse manager, a head nurse and a psychiatric nurse.

Triage Course. The BCH ED has an extensive advanced triage system. The system operates 24 hours a day, with one or two nurses assigned to triage for each shift. The nurses' primary responsibility is to categorize the nature and severity of a patient's illness and determine where and how soon the patient should be seen. The nurses are allowed to refer patients to clinic when the clinic is open. They also request certain diagnostic tests (primarily extremity x-rays) from triage when this will expedite a patient's release. The triage assignment is busy, challenging and stressful.

A few months after orientation, nurses are provided with a triage course. The course is one and one-half days long and focuses on initial assessment of common illnesses and injuries. Topics covered include:

- the role of the triage nurse
- stress in triage
- chest pain
- orthopaedic complaints and x-ray requests
- neurologic triage
- abdominal pain
- obstetric/gynaecologic triage
- paediatric triage
- psychiatric triage

Faculty include the clinical nurse specialist, nurse manager, a head nurse, psychiatric nurse, clinical nurses and physicians.

CEDNEP. CEDNEP is a standardized statewide specialty education programme for emergency nurses, directed by nursing staff at the Massachusetts Office of Emergency Medical Services. Approximately 1700 nurses have attended the course since its inception in 1976. The course has become the educational standard for Massachusetts emergency nurses, and most EDs attempt to have all staff attend the programme.

CEDNEP is about 110 hours in length. It covers medical, surgical, traumatic, paediatric and psychiatric emergencies, and is taught mostly by nurses. The course objectives state that, at the completion of the programme, the participant will be able to:

- 'describe the Emergency Medical Services System (EMSS), including the capabilities of pre-hospital personnel, communication and transfer protocols/procedures
- demonstrate support for the EMSS through participation on state/regional EMS committees, planning/lecturing for CEDNEP and other educational programmes sponsored by EMS agencies
- describe the professional and clinical role/responsibilities of the emergency nurse
- demonstrate professional development through research, education of self/peers/students/community membership on committees, and writing for/reviewing the literature' (Capasso, Kelley and Halkola 1983:2).

CEDNEP itself is supplemented by the two-day Advanced Cardiac Life Support course (American Heart Association 1983) focusing on emergency cardiac care. In addition to the didactic content, nurses spend one day each observing with an ambulance service and in a selected clinical facility (ED, burn unit, spinal cord injury centre).

CEDNEP is offered several times a year across the state. One or two hospitals host each programme for emergency nurses in their area. BCH has hosted CEDNEP several times, and several of the nursing staff serve as faculty.

BCH TNC. In 1984, the ED received a grant from the Massachusetts Office of Emergency Medical Services to develop a trauma nurse course. Thus far our course has been presented several times in various parts of the state. The TNC is coordinated by the clinical nurse specialist and nurse manager and taught entirely by BCH ED nurses.

The BCH TNC is a two-day programme for emergency nurses intended to improve knowledge and skills related to care of the trauma patient. Lecture topics include assessment, head, chest or abdominal trauma, orthopaedic injuries, paediatric trauma, psycho-trauma, trauma epidemiology and principles of team resuscitation. The programme also includes demonstration and practice sessions for technical skills such as the use of anti-shock trousers, autotransfusion and airway management. The course concludes with demonstration, practice and testing in the Mega-Trauma station. In this station, the student is exposed to three different simulated patient scenarios. Working with moulaged victims, students are expected to correctly assess injuries and describe appropriate treatment. Mega-Trauma is very educational and also a lot of fun!

3.4.6 Recognition of excellence

(a) *Overview*

Recent management literature (Peters and Austin 1985; Peters and Waterman 1982; Smith, Reinow and Reid 1984; Younger 1983) has highlighted a change in emphasis from technical to interpersonal skills. The concept of 'productivity through people' (Peters and Waterman 1982) suggests that happy employees are productive employees, and productive employees are the key to a successful enterprise.

The major tenets of this management philosophy (Peters and Austin 1985; Peters and Waterman 1982) are to respect the individual, treat people as adults and make people winners. The company is viewed as an extended family and this view is expressed through a genuine 'people orientation', an emphasis on positive reinforcement, informal style and use of small teams. The company's goals are stated explicitly and their achievement is celebrated with 'hoopla, celebration, and verve'.

Hoopla, celebration and verve signify the creation of a work setting that stimulates enthusiasm, in which 'everybody wins regularly'. The intent is to reward performance with multiple positive reinforcements. Contests, awards and games, tee-shirts and mottos, newsletters and posters, parties and banquets may all be used to produce such an environment. The method may seem silly but it is effective and the outcome is a positive emphasis on goals and goal achievement.

(b) *Implementation*

The nursing leadership decided to create a recognition award in order to increase the opportunity for positive reinforcement of staff. The night head nurse chaired a task force to discuss the award, and it was decided that the award would recognize excellence in clinical nursing. Nurses would be nominated on the basis of several criteria which included:

- employment of at least six months duration
- CEDNEP or CEN credentials
- emergency nursing clinical expertise
- serving as a role model to colleagues
- contribution to ED professional activities as a preceptor or teacher
- charge nurse or committee member

A selection committee composed of staff and management would choose one nurse to receive the award. The winner would receive a plaque and a small sum of money to be used for educational purposes. All qualified candidates would receive recognition.

At the time of this writing, the criteria had been established, with the nomination and selection process yet to occur. It is hoped that the award will be viewed positively by the nursing staff as a recognition of their excellence. The leadership plans to develop other positive reinforcements after the award process is completed.

3.4.7 Patient classification

(a) *Overview*

Patient classification systems (PCSs) are becoming a necessity in US EDs. A PCS classifies patients by acuity, defines the nursing time required for each type of patient and specifies the number of nursing staff required to care for a given number of patients. In addition to being required by JCAH (1984), these systems provide an objective method of justifying staffing and thus are helpful in countering cost-control pressures.

PCSs were originally developed for use in in-patient wards. There are a few packaged systems available for sale, but many hospitals develop their own because even the packaged systems must be adapted to the hospital's unique characteristics. Buschiazzo (1984a, 1984b), Kromash (1984), and Schulmerich (1984) have all described their ED PCSs but these packaged systems are not yet generally available.

There are two types of classification instruments: prototype and factor (Giovannetti 1979). In the prototype format, several categories of acuity are delineated according to general descriptions of patient characteristics, and an individual patient is placed in the one category where he best fits. In the factor format, several factors or subcategories of acuity are delineated rather than just one category. A patient is placed where he best fits in each factor, scores for each factor are totalled, and the patient is categorized by total score. The factor instrument is more accurate but the prototype instrument is easier, which may be why it has been used for all the present ED PCSs.

(b) *Implementation*

In Boston, a group of ED nurse managers decided to pool their efforts and develop a PCS jointly. This project by a subcommittee of the regional emergency medical services nursing committee began in early 1985.

The process is very tedious and our system is still being developed, but there will probably be six categories, based on the amount of nursing time required. The levels are minimal, moderate, comprehensive, intensive, maximal and exceptional. Patients will be placed into a category according to their classification by physiologic stability, technical interventions, mobility, communications/knowledge and psychosocial status. Whether the instrument will be factor or prototype has yet to be resolved.

Direct and indirect nursing activities and nonproductive time will all be measured. Nonproductive time includes paid time off, educational, committee, and administrative time. Indirect activities, which include tasks like ordering medication stock, checking and stocking equipment and supplies, rounds and telephone calls, were analysed early in 1986. The classification instrument was beginning to be tested, preparatory to time and motion studies in the various departments.

The group process in a project of this type has both advantages and disadvantages. The disadvantages are that the process is more time-consuming and each member of the group may have to make compromises. The advantages are the increased support provided by a group, more thoughtful and comprehensive deliberations, built-in expert validity and a product that will have multi-hospital applicability.

CONCLUSION

The practice of emergency nursing is constantly changing. Sometimes it is disconcerting to contemplate the difficulties of keeping up with new developments. And yet, mastering change and uncertainty is an emergency nurse's forte.

This chapter has described the efforts of one ED to master the challenges of change and uncertainty at the departmental level. The tools used were knowledge of current trends in emergency nursing, assessment of the ED's unique strengths and weaknesses and a systematic management approach. The results were the professional development of the nursing staff and the introduction of programmes that fostered excellence in emergency nursing.

ACKNOWLEDGEMENT

The author would like to acknowledge the assistance of the leadership team (Joseph Blansfield, RN, MS, CEN, Clinical Nurse Specialist; S. Lindsay Boyd Bringhurst, RN, CEN, Clinical Coordinator; James

Chaisson, RN, CEN, Evening Head Nurse; Patricia Maher, RN, CEN, Night Head Nurse) and the clinical nursing staff, without whom these activities could not have been accomplished.

EDITOR'S NOTES

The use of standardized assessment routines is not the only factor used to reduce error rates: major accident centres mean patients are being treated at specialist centres. The benefits of this centralization are well known, as D. D. Trunkey (1983) indicates in relating his experiences in the US (see Further Reading). Advances in nursing practice and roles are discussed by Steve Wright (1985) (see Further Reading).

In our department, we used to have a joke that when you returned from two weeks' holiday you needed some retraining because of the rapid changes that occur in emergency nursing. This can be very stimulating, but it may also leave you feeling inadequate and ill-informed. This chapter's sections on practice, management, and professional development focus on some important issues of practice.

Diane Danis's comprehensive list of references must fulfil every editor's long-held wishes. My only additions, other than the ones mentioned, explore possibilities of expanded family participation and suggestions to help the patient maintain contact with reality.

REFERENCES

American College of Emergency Physicians (1983) Emergency care guidelines. In Emergency Department Nurses Association, *Standards of emergency nursing practice*, (Mosby, St. Louis, MO, pp. 96–106 (reprinted from *Annals of Emergency Medicine* (1982) **11**, 222–26).

American Heart Association (1983) *Textbook of Advanced Cardiac Life Support*. American Heart Association, Dallas.

American Nurses Association (1980) *Nursing: A Social Policy Statement*. American Nurses Association, Kansas City, MO.

Bell, M.L. (1980) Management by objectives. *Journal of Nursing Administration*, **10**(5), 19–26.

Blansfield, J., Fackler, C., and Bergeron, K. (1985) Developing standardized care plans: One emergency department's experience. *Journal of Emergency Nursing*, **11**, 304–9.

Buschiazzo, L. (1984a) Patient classification in the emergency department.

Letter to the editor. *Journal of Emergency Nursing*, **10**, 7–8.

Buschiazzo, L. (1984b) Patient classification in the emergency department. Letter to the editor. *Journal of Emergency Nursing*, **10**, 183–4.

Capasso, V.C., Kelley, S.J., and Halkola, P.M. (1983) *Curriculum of the Critical-Care Emergency Department Nurse Education Program* (2nd edn). Department of Public Health, Boston, MA.

Cousins, A. (1984) Management of the ED patient with a borderline personality disorder. *Journal of Emergency Nursing*, **10**, 94–6.

Deegan, A.X., and O'Donovan, T.R. (1982) *Management by Objectives for Hospitals* (2nd edn). Aspen, Rockville, MD.

Drucker, P.F. (1954) *The Practice of Management*. Harper & Row, New York.

Emergency Department Nurses Association (now Emergency Nurses Association) (1983) *Standards of Emergency Nursing Practice*. Mosby, St. Louis, MO.

Emergency Department Nurse Association (now Emergency Nurses Association) (1985) *Core curriculum* (2nd edn). Saunders, Philadelphia, PA (originally published 1980).

Frank, I.C. and McGovern, F. (1983) Marketing one hospital's emergency department. *Journal of Emergency Nursing*, **9**, 324–6.

Giovannetti, P. (1979) Understanding patient classification systems. *The Journal of Nursing Administration*, **8**(2), 4–9.

Heister, K., Johnson, B., and Trimberger, L. (1982) ED standards and audit criteria. *Journal of Emergency Nursing*, **8**, 83–7.

Joint Commission on Accreditation of Hospitals (1984) *Accreditation Manual for Hospitals*. Joint Commission on Accreditation of Hospitals, Chicago.

Kromash, E.J. (1984) Patient classification and required nursing time in a pediatric emergency department. *Journal of Emergency Nursing*, **10**, 69–73.

Murphy, J.G. and Jacobson, S. (1984) Assessing the quality of emergency care: The medical record versus patient outcome. *Annals of Emergency Medicine*, **13**, 158–65.

Neff, J. (1985) Abdominal pain, gastrointestinal bleeding, and orthopedic injury. *Journal of Emergency Nursing*, **11**, 339–44.

Peters, T. and Austin, N. (1985) *A Passion for Excellence: The Leadership Difference*. Random House, New York.

Peters, T.J. and Waterman, R.H. (1982) *In Search of Excellence: Lessons From America's Best-Run Companies*. Warner, New York.

Pollock, C.S. (1983) Adapting management by objectives to nursing. *Nursing Clinics of North America*, **18**, 481–90.

Rich, C. (1982) Special Needs Kardex: An answer for repeaters. *Journal of Emergency Nursing*, **8**, 191–5.

Schulmerich, S.C. (1984) Developing a patient classification system for the emergency department. *Journal of Emergency Nursing*, **10**, 298–305.

Smith, H.L., Reinow, F.D., and Reid, R.A. (1984) Japanese management: Implications for nursing administration. *The Journal of Nursing Administration*, **14**, 33–9.

Thompson, J.D. (1984) Evolving trends in emergency nursing. In J.G. Parker (ed.), *Emergency Nursing: A Guide to Comprehensive Care*, Wiley, New York, pp. 595–604.

Vestal, K.W. (1984) Marketing concepts for the emergency department. *Journal of Emergency Nursing*, **10**, 274–6.

Walts, L. and Blair, F. (1983) Making quality assurance work in the emergency department. *Journal of Emergency Nursing*, **9**, 59–60.

Younger, J.B. (1983) Theory Z management and health care organizations. *Nursing Economics*, **1**, 40–5, 69.

FURTHER READING

Doyle, C., Pool, H., Burrey, R.E. et al. (1987) Family participation during resuscitation: An option. *Annals of Emergency Medicine*, **16**, 6.

Murant, J.E., Hurten, N., and Mesny, J. (1985) The use of standardised assessment procedures in the evaluation of patients in multiple injuries. *Archives of Emergency Medicine*, **2**, 11.

Nichol, K.A. (1984) *Psychological Care in Physical Illness*. Croom Helm, London.

Stratton, H. (1981) Keeping the patient in touch with reality. *Care of the Critically Ill*, **3**, 1.

Trunkey, D.D. (1983) Trauma. *Scientific American*, **20**, 7.

Wright, S. (1985) New nurses: new boundaries. *Nursing Practice*, **1**, 1

4

Provision of Pre-Hospital Care

Gary J. Jones

The provision of pre-hospital care in this country primarily rests with the ambulance service. This, however, does not apply to all countries. In the US most pre-hospital care is provided by the fire department, though some states use the police, voluntary groups, and in a few, a recognized third emergency service that can be compared to the acute activities of British ambulance services. Many countries on the continent use medical and nursing teams as the first line response; in France the system of medical and nursing teams that respond to the scene of accidents or sudden illness is called Société d'Assistance Medicale Urgence (SAMU). This system is based on districts. Each district is given a SAMU number and the complete system is based at the district hospital.

Thus, the provision of pre-hospital care is varied and depends on many factors such as the country and area of work. This chapter will deal primarily with the nursing practice and management of pre-hospital care both in this county and abroad. It will deal with education for, and actual provision of, care by the nurse and pre-hospital colleagues. Nurses' attitudes, job description and local policy all affect the impact nurses can have on pre-hospital care.

Nurses working in Accident and Emergency departments come into contact with ambulance personnel on a daily basis, yet the extent of the nurses' knowledge of the ambulance service is often sparse. Unless the nurse has first-hand experience of the pre-hospital care, attitudes and lack of knowledge can often influence views on the care provided.

4.1 HISTORY OF THE BRITISH AMBULANCE SERVICE

Prior to 1948 local authorities were not obligated to provide an ambulance service. Much of the transport was provided by the Red Cross and St. John ambulances. During the Second World War, Civil Defence provided many of the ambulances needed to transport injured civilians to hospital. With the National Health Service Act of 1946, the local authority became responsible for providing ambulance transport, as enacted in 1948. Ambulance crews were basically untrained and even up until the late 1960s required only a valid first aid certificate from the Voluntary Aid Societies. Much of the care provided was 'scoop and run' (Easton 1977).

Ambulance training is now highly organized and controlled through a National Staff Council. Care is provided on site and patients are transported, when stable, to the hospital. All first line emergency vehicles are staffed by fully trained personnel. A six-week ambulance aid training course is provided at regional training schools. The student must also spend one year in service before being allowed to undertake emergency calls with junior staff. More senior ambulance crews are now being offered advanced training in life support to enable the best care to be provided at the scene.

A major difference between the ambulance service in Britain and the US is the lack of on-site communication to the hospital in this country. In the US, paramedics are linked to base hospitals and establish a radio link between the accident scene and hospital when dealing with patients. Advice and control of the incident is provided by medical or nursing personnel. In Britain, advanced trained crews (paramedics) work within strict protocols but diagnose and treat without reference to a hospital.

4.2 ON-SITE MEDICAL AND NURSING CARE

With advanced training and knowledge more care can be provided by ambulance staff; however, there will still be a need in some instances for medical and nursing intervention in the pre-hospital setting. At present two major systems exist in Britain to provide this extra care: the general practitioner-based schemes established by the British Association for Immediate Care, and hospital-based schemes.

GP-based schemes began in the mid-1960s and were formally

organized and operational in December 1967. The founder of this scheme, which now stretches throughout Britain, was Ken Easton, a Yorkshire GP. He recognized the need for medical aid at road accidents and provided such care as required. Emergency services supported this innovation and now medical presence in many situations is an accepted part of pre-hospital care (Easton 1977).

Hospital teams are usually resourced by the Accident and Emergency Department, although if the team is primarily used for pre-hospital cardiac care it will be organized from the Coronary Care Unit. Accident response teams can be subdivided into day-to-day mobile teams and teams that respond only to a major incident.

4.2.1 Twenty-four hour mobile teams

Twenty-four hour mobile teams provide medical and nursing care to the few victims whose immediate transportation to hospital is not advisable or whose entrapment prevents movement. The team usually consists of one doctor and one nurse, although this will vary according to local needs. Not all hospitals provide such teams and areas where neither a hospital nor GP scheme exists have no means of on-site medical or nursing care.

Call out of teams is usually initiated by the ambulance service, although local arrangements may allow for other entities to activate the system. Two types of call out are the blanket and selected call. In a blanket call out system, the emergency services mobilize the hospital team on receiving an emergency call prior to the arrival on scene of the ambulance crew. In a selected call, the ambulance crew on arrival will summon the team if required. Although there is merit to both methods, the selected call controls the indiscriminate mobilization of medical and nursing teams.

The hospital unit travels to the scene either by use of a hospital-based emergency vehicle or by the local ambulance or police service. If a specific emergency vehicle is used, it will normally be owned by the hospital. This vehicle may be a converted ambulance or a Landrover, depending on local requirements and the type of intervention necessary. Derby Royal Infirmary provide emergency vehicles of the Landrover type which are fully equipped and used to transport the team to the scene. Patients are transported in a local authority ambulance. Other hospitals using a converted ambulance will transport the patient within their own vehicle. Again, there are advantages and disadvantages with both methods and each hospital must evaluate both before making a decision. Mobilization of an on-site vehicle prevents delay but the provision of drivers and parking facilities may deter many authorities. The use of emergency service vehicles and personnel reduces cost but the amount of equipment taken to the scene and its storage must be considered carefully, with easy access a paramount consideration.

4.2.2 Equipment

Because of the need for easy access and carrying, equipment taken to the scene must be both light and sturdy enough to withstand being knocked and dropped. The chosen container must allow clear identification of all equipment. It is pointless to have to delve into a bottomless box of equipment at the roadside. Since the hospital cannot go to the patient, it is unnecessary to try to bring along all of its equipment. What is needed is equipment to support life functions and the relief of pain (Easton 1977). Equipment essential for restoring and maintaining vital functions is listed below.

(a) *Respiratory care*

Respiratory care requires the use of Guedal airways, portable suction equipment, intubation equipment, a bag and mask, and an emergency tracheostomy set. Having a clear airway may be sufficient for normal breathing; however, should a tension pneumothorax develop, a chest drain and Heimlich Valve will allow for immediate intervention.

Ventilation can be provided by a resuscitation bag but it may be easier to use a portable ventilator; Pneupack and Motivus are two such systems.

(b) *Circulation*

Volume replacement can be provided for trauma victims by many infusion solutions such as Haemacell. Whichever solution is used should be transported in plastic bottles — glass bottles in the pre-hospital setting can be disastrous.

Other essential equipment are large-bore IV cannula to facilitate the infusion of colloids and blood or other fluids (e.g. size 14E), drugs required in the event of cardiac arrest and a selected anti-arrhythmia drug. A portable monitor/defibrillator is also a necessary part of pre-hospital care of the cardiovascular system.

(c) *Pain relief*

Pain relief requires the use of Entonox, narcotic drugs and non-narcotic analgesics. The use of analgesics in the pre-hospital setting is essential although particular care must be maintained with patients whose state of consciousness requires regular monitoring, for example, because of the nature of their injuries. The use of sedatives is also helpful at the site.

Other items to be included are a hard cervical collar (e.g. Hines) if one is not provided by the ambulance service; a dextrose IV for use with the hypoglycaemic patient; Narcan to reverse the analgesia if necessary; and clips, blades and sutures to establish intravenous infusions and tying of vessels if necessary.

(d) *Protective clothing*

Staff must be protected from environmental hazards when working in the pre-hospital site. It is quite wrong to expect nurses to crawl under cars in dresses and caps: waterproof suits with adequate insulation must be worn. These suits must be reflective to prevent injury from moving vehicles at the scene of an accident. Helmets are vital as many road accidents can be fatal to a nurse with an unprotected head. Boots must be worn and trouser legs must not be pushed inside the boots (to prevent corrosive chemicals running down inside boots). Where necessary, gloves and goggles should be available so that the nurse is well protected and warm.

4.3 ORGANIZATION OF A 24-HOUR RESPONSE TEAM

Because such a team must be available 24 hours per day, it is essential that staffing arrangements allow a doctor and nurse to be released from the department at any time. All staff appointed to such a department must be willing to participate in pre-hospital care, and the job description should reflect this agreement. Insurance coverage for injury to individuals must be organized through the health authority. This insurance is usually provided in a separate agreement with the insurance company.

Adequate equipment and clothing must be provided, and readily accessible storage facilities arranged. Regular checking and replacement of equipment and clothes should be carried out by the nursing staff. This regular check also continually updates the nurses' awareness of the equipment carried and its availability. Equipment should be stored in bags or small cases for ease in use. The bags or cases should be waterproof, and open and close easily. Large boxes are not easy to use in the type of situations the team may be called to, and are useless if left open while dealing with patients during a snowstorm.

Staff training is essential. Ideally, a new doctor or nurse should go as an observer for the first few calls, but this will depend on staffing levels and time of call. Clothing and boots should be tried before a call, as nothing is more disruptive than a new nurse or doctor trying on boots that are too large or small while the vehicle is waiting.

Mobilization will depend on local methods. If the emergency vehicle and drivers are in the hospital, an adequate paging system will be needed to facilitate deployment. If a service vehicle is used, it must be organized through the ambulance or police service. Equipment must be removed from storage and prepared to go into the ambulance or police car on arrival.

It is essential when mobilizing the team to remember the patients within the department. Where necessary, adequate handover to other staff is important and no disruption to the care of patients in the department should occur when the team is mobilized. A senior nurse should remain within the department to prepare resuscitation areas and maintain control of the unit.

Staff providing the pre-hospital care should be experienced; where cardiac care is provided the staff should be experienced Coronary Care Unit nurses and doctors. Staff members must remember that their role is to provide life support and pain relief. As soon as the patient is sufficiently stable, he or she should be moved to hospital with all due care and speed.

4.3.1 The nurses' role in the 24-hour team

The role the nurse plays in pre-hospital care depends very much on the type of care required. A cardiac patient may well have a mobile coronary care unit arrive from the local hospital. For example, the Belfast Coronary Care ambulance and team is provided from the Royal Victoria Hospital. This unit responds to all calls from GPs or ambulance crews whose patients are suffering chest pain. A nurse and doctor from the Coronary Care Unit respond in an ambulance fully equipped with a stretcher, monitor/defibrillator and IV solutions. Drugs and intubation and back-up equipment are provided within the vehicle in some cases. Radio communication between the ambulance and the Coronary Care Unit is available. The local ambulance service drive the vehicle to the hospital to collect the team.

The patient is stabilized at home or in the street and then transported to hospital. The nurse, highly trained in coronary care nursing, responds not only to the immediate clinical needs of the patient but can also begin the psychological care this person will require on the way to recovery. This care can be administered by the Accident and Emergency nurse to a person trapped in a vehicle. The patient suffering multiple injuries needs both physical and psychological care which can begin at the accident scene with the nurse providing holistic care throughout.

Normally the patient from a road traffic accident will be treated by many professionals, all fragmenting the care. With pre-hospital care from a hospital-based team, holistic care can begin as the nurse follows the patient from the incident scene to the department and on to the minor theatre or ward. On arrival at the scene the nurse is able to assess the total situation — the type and method of injury, and patient response. The exact physical and psychological trauma can be assessed and anticipated at this early stage. Actual and potential problems can be identified and goals set. Short-term goals can be achieved at the scene with rapid intervention. These short-term goals mainly include stabilization of airway, breathing and circulation. Intervention requires an explanation to the patient of what is to be done and, as necessary and possible, support of the relatives. Long-term goals for the accident room and beyond can be organized.

Intervention on site will depend on the patient's condition, but a rapport with the patient can be developed throughout the duration of the pre-hospital setting, later continuing into the department. This relationship between patient and nurse could never be provided without nurses in the pre-hospital field. Evaluation is made much easier when the nurse has dealt with the patient from the very onset. Because of good pre-hospital care by ambulance staff many nurses do not see patients in the same condition as they were found at the scene. Inability to assess the patient's situation until arrival at hospital leaves the nurse with a large gap when attempting evaluation. The nurse at the scene, having followed the patient throughout both the pre-hospital and in-hospital care, can avoid this gap and make a much more valuable evaluation of the patient. The achievement of goals set on arrival at the scene and for in-hospital care can be more easily evaluated.

4.3.2 Communication from site to base

Good communication between the team on site and the Accident and Emergency Department or Coronary Care Unit is essential. By radio link the team can update the nursing staff within the department to make specific preparation for the arrival. Establishment of a base radio within the hospital department is therefore important as it allows a link between the site and hospital. Portable radios are often useful on site if the patient is a distance from the ambulance or emergency vehicle (Caroline 1979).

4.3.3 Records

Keeping records is a valuable and necessary part of pre-hospital care. The record form should be easy to use and as brief as possible. Only essential information such as the patients' vital signs, assessment of the situation and interventions need be recorded. If blood specimens are sent to the hospital for crossmatch, adequate records with personal identification numbers must be used. Blood labelled with the patient's record number can be sent to hospital with the police, and crossmatched blood will then be available on arrival. A wristband showing the record number should be attached to the patient.

4.3.4 Advanced life support and the nurse

Much controversy surrounds the extended role of the nurse. Departments vary greatly as to the procedures nurses may undertake. Within the pre-hospital setting there is often a need for the nurse to be able to perform advanced life support. Two patients, in separate cars in an accident, may both need advanced life support. If the nurse is unable to perform such skills, then her ability to support each patient's life functions is diminished. Some hospitals that provide 24-hour teams specifically allow nurses, after in-service education, to perform such skills as intravenous cannulation, intubation and defibrillation. Without such skills the effectiveness of nursing care at the scene may be diminished.

4.4 FIVE HOURS AT THE SCENE

This true story describes how medical and nursing personnel became a part of the pre-hospital care team in a department that provides a 24-hour response.

Just before 6:00 a.m. in midsummer the emergency bleep was activated by the switchboard to call the Sister of the Accident Department at Orsett Hospital. Ambulance control asked for a mobile team to attend a road accident in which a lorry driver was trapped. After collecting the team's equipment and putting on protective clothing the doctor and nurse left the department in a county ambulance.

On arrival at scene, the lorry was seen to be turned over and down a grass slope. The rescue was made more difficult by a previous accident only days before that had left the area covered in manure. Although the driver was trapped by his legs and lower body, he was conscious and breathing well. An intravenous infusion of Haemacell was commenced rapidly and a second infusion was sited with great difficulty. Support for the patient's neck and upper body was provided.

The position of entrapment caused great difficulty for removal. The only method that could be employed was to dismantle the cab and, with heavy lifting and winching equipment, pull the engine and front of the cab away from the driver. This took some hours during which intravenous analgesia was given.

At 9:00 a.m. the team was changed and the nurse and doctor brought back to the department so that they could go off duty. The driver's condition was becoming much worse; blood was sent from the scene for crossmatched and non-crossmatched O negative blood. Blood transfusion then began.

At 10:00 a.m. when the clinical assistant and I attended the scene, the intravenous lines were giving cause for concern so a cut down provided much more stable access to the venous system. The driver by this time had been heavily sedated with intravenous analgesia and sedatives. Before release the crossmatched blood was available and sent to the scene.

Just before 10:30 a.m. the driver was released. When he arrived in the Accident Department at 11:00 a.m., he had a blood pressure of 130/60 and a pulse rate of 85.

This case shows that pre-hospital care can stabilize a patient even after lengthy entrapment. The nurse in this situation was able to remain with the patient throughout much of his ordeal. Although there was a need to replace the nurse at one point, the second nurse was able to follow the driver through his care until admission to the theatre.

The nurse was responsible for all equipment at the scene, up-to-date recording of vital signs and treatment administered. The nurse was able to provide the link between the patient and the other emergency services on site. When relatives arrived at the hospital the nurse was able to spend time with them discussing the ordeal the driver had undergone. This was a great help to the relatives, who had the advantage of talking to a nurse who had actually been at the scene and nursed the driver throughout much of the time since the accident.

4.5 PRE-HOSPITAL CARE IN A MAJOR INCIDENT

All Accident and Emergency Departments should be able to respond to the need for pre-hospital care at the scene of a major incident. As in the case of a department that provides a day-to-day cover, the equipment and clothing intended for coping with major incidents must be easy to use, correctly stored and regularly checked. Equipment is essentially the same as described earlier; however, there will be a need for much more equipment to be transported to the scene. This transportation may be difficult if dozens of small bags or boxes are taken. At Orsett Accident and Emergency Department, the major incident equipment is stored in large boxes that can be lifted by one person. Six small shoulder bags are taken which contain dressings, intravenous infusion and airway equipment. The large boxes would be held at the casualty clearing station of the incident and used both for restocking the shoulder bags and within the casualty clearing area.

The role of the nurse in a major incident is different from that of a nurse in the day-to-day mobile team. Although care will be provided in the pre-hospital setting, a one-to-one relationship with the patient will not be possible because of the number of patients involved. Nurses should primarily work at the casualty clearing station, where there will be a need to hold many injured persons until transportation to hospital can be arranged. The nurses need to establish an Accident and Emergency Department on site. Equipment will be limited and the nurse must bring all her knowledge and skills to the fore. Ambulance and fire crews will transport the patients to the clearing station. Where patients are trapped, nurses and medical staff may be asked to move into the area and provide care prior to release. Here the nurse would make use of the shoulder bags for easy access to equipment and drugs.

4.5.1 Control of the nursing team

The size of the accident and number of injured persons will often determine the number of nurses required. Most teams usually mobilize four to six nurses but this will vary. A senior nurse from the Accident Department must take charge of this team and liaise with the site medical officer and other incident officers. It must be made clear to all nurses present that they follow only the senior nurse's orders and directions. Other professionals must use the senior nurse as the link between themselves and nurses on site. It is the responsibility of the senior nurse to provide nurses either at the clearing station or for patient care at the scene. A record of nurses within the disaster area must be maintained to eliminate the possibility of loss of staff due to injury.

Many patients may arrive at the casualty clearing station and they must be nursed as within the temporary Accident and Emergency Department until transported to hospital. The senior nurse must keep track of all equipment and not allow other personnel to remove it indiscriminately.

Nurses will become fatigued and regular change of nursing teams is important. The pre-hospital team should be replaced after approximately two hours; particularly in cold weather when hypothermia may well begin to develop.

4.5.2 Triage

Because of the number of people injured, an organized system of care and evacuation to hospital — triage — must exist. Each injured person is assessed for injuries and urgency of care. Depending on the need an urgency rating will be given. The most common system is the three-rating system: immediate, urgent and delayed. If a patient is in need of resuscitation and life support a rating of 'immediate' will be given. If seriously injured but in no need of immediate resuscitation an urgent rating is given. A delayed rating is given to those with less severe injuries or injuries that cannot be treated.

The rating given is identified by the use of cards attached to the patient. Colour coding also helps to facilitate the identification of whom to treat or transport next. We use red cards for immediate treatment, yellow for urgent and green to signify delayed treatment. Anyone who dies at the scene will also be labelled accordingly and left to one side until all casualties are dealt with.

As soon as possible the 'immediate' patients will be transported to hospital. These patients may require nursing intervention en route. The senior nurse, in consultation with the medical officer, must decide if nursing escorts are necessary. The staff on site must not be depleted if at all possible.

4.5.3 Preparation for major incidents

Each hospital providing emergency facilities should have a major incident plan. Included in this plan will usually be a mobile team. In past disasters many problems have arisen because medical and nursing teams were collected and sent off unaware of their role or the equipment available. If the hospital is receiving patients from the incident it is very difficult to send all experienced Accident and Emergency staff to the scene. The plan for disasters should therefore include nurses from acute wards. These nurses should be under the direction of the senior nurse as previously described. A sufficient number of nurses should be pre-designated for such an event and spend time on a regular basis familiarizing themselves with the equipment. Nurses from acute wards like their A and E colleagues, should be aware of the correct clothing, boots and helmet to wear.

The site medical officer is the most senior doctor at the scene. Many plans differ in the rank and position of this person. Some plans designate a consultant, others a senior registrar, a gynaecologist, physician, surgeon, or the Accident and Emergency consultant. Whoever is sent should have an in-depth knowledge of pre-hospital care, the organization of medical services, and needs at the site of a major accident. Where GP schemes exist, it is a good idea to include these people in the major incident plan, as they often have more experience of pre-hospital care and handling disasters than most hospital-based doctors.

The medical and nursing staff involved in a major incident are in alien territory. The comfort of a warm, well-lit, well-equipped department is gone. Emergency services can and will be a great help if asked. It is important to remember that they are in their usual environment and know the pitfalls. Liaison with all services when setting up and updating plans aids better patient care and safety for staff.

4.6 THE NURSE AND PRE-HOSPITAL CARE IN THE US

Many areas of the US enjoy highly advanced pre-hospital care carried out by paramedic personnel. Each state in the US varies greatly in the degree of influence nurses have in the pre-hospital setting. In California the nurse's role in caring for the pre-hospital patient is immense. Not only do nurses control much of the training but they also control calls from paramedics within the department.

When a paramedic crew arrives on scene, state law dictates that they must radio the hospital, present information about their patient and carry out care following instructions by radio from the staff within the base hospital's Emergency Department. In many states only registered medical practitioners may control calls. However, in California state law allows nurses who are certified by the state to undertake control of the calls.

The paramedic will follow the nurse's instructions with regard to administration of drugs, intravenous infusion and other methods of intervention. The nurse has a responsibility to obtain a clear history and assessment of each patient. From this history the nurse will make a decision as to the treatment required. The nurse will require updates of vital signs, general condition after treatment, and will decide when it is safe to transport the patient. Electrocardiogram recordings will be sent via telemetry and the nurse will interpret these and advise treatment for the present arrhythmia. To undertake such a responsibility the nurse must understand the pre-hospital situation. As a part of the nurse's training for this position she will accompany the paramedics for several weeks to learn their problems and difficulties. This enables the nurse, when in radio control, to appreciate the environment and visualize the situation. A two-week course is also a mandatory part of this training. The nurse undertaking this course must be registered in advanced life support and work actively within the Emergency Department. On completion of the course and pre-hospital care trips the nurse is awarded the state MICN certificate (Mobile Intensive Care Nurse).

4.6.1 Observation of an MICN taking a call

The bell rang and a light flashed indicating a radio call from a paramedic unit that required attention. The charge nurse entered the radio room and established contact with a paramedic crew at Los Angeles International Airport treating a male patient in cardiac arrest.

The patient was in asystole. The crew sent an electrocardiograph (ECG) strip via telemetry; the nurse instructed the crew to intubate and give various drugs after starting an intravenous infusion. When further ECG tracings showed ventricular fibrillation, instruction to defibrillate was given by the nurse and Lignocaine was ordered.

Information from the paramedic crew then indicated that femoral pulses were present and sinus tachycardia was shown on the ECG. The nurse ordered the crew to transport the patient, who arrived several minutes later with good peripheral pulses.

The call was recorded and logged as it occurred. The report was signed and made ready for the liaison nurse to review.

4.7 EDUCATING NON-NURSING PERSONNEL FOR PRE-HOSPITAL CARE

Nurses have a very important role to play in the education of other pre-hospital personnel. This involvement should cover the total spectrum of basic through advanced training. In order to involve nurses in this education, they must be prepared to advance their own knowledge and skills and then participate in the training of the pre-hospital care-givers. Nursing involvement is best seen in the training of fire department personnel in paramedic skills throughout the US. Not all states have programmes that actively involve nurses, but even where the nurses are not actively involved with the programme or lectures, they still play a vital role in training fire department personnel within the Emergency Department.

Within the state of California, nurses are certified by the county to act as paramedic liaison nurses. These nurses are responsible for organizing hospital paramedic training, continued education, and reviewing all tapes and logs of paramedic calls. In paramedic training schools the administration and teaching of paramedics is primarily the responsibility of nurses. These nurses, like the liaison nurse, are certified by the county to carry out this training.

In Britain nurses are becoming more involved with ambulance training although the majority of education is provided by the service's own instructors. Nurses can participate actively as guest lecturers for basic and refresher training.

With the advent of advanced training for ambulance personnel, nurses from Accident and Emergency Departments will become more involved with in-service training and with the programmes and education of our pre-hospital colleagues.

4.8 ADVANCED TRAINING OF AMBULANCE SERVICES IN BRITAIN

An agreement has been reached that a national package will be available for advanced training of ambulance personnel in life support skills such as intubation, intravenous cannulation, defibrillation and drug administration. This is called *Extended Training in Ambulance Aid*, by the Ambulance Staff Training Committee (published by the NHS Training Authority, Bristol). It will require lectures to be provided at ambulance training schools and in-service training within hospitals. This training will be held in operating theatres, Accident Departments and Coronary Care Units. Nurses must become involved with this training and therefore must become educated themselves about pre-hospital care.

Nursing staff from Coronary Care Units and Accident Departments have a great wealth of knowledge to impart to the ambulance staff, especially with regard to continuous care of patients. Pre-hospital personnel are very good at assessment but advanced skills require further education in continuous evaluation of patients and the need to respond with treatment to a patient's changing condition.

The correct treatment of a patient suffering a cardiac condition requires teaching by a nurse. To treat correctly a patient with multiple injuries in the pre-hospital period usually requires an experienced A and E nurse, but the required skills can be conveyed to ambulance personnel. If nurses do not become involved, there will be a gap in patient care because treatment will be neglected in the period immediately after injury or the onset of illness.

Advanced training for ambulance personnel has been operating for some years under the Association of Emergency Medical Technicians (AEMT) and local authorities. Only recently has the national package been agreed. Most AEMT and local authority schemes have had a high input from nursing staff. Avon ambulance service advanced training, for example, has engaged the nursing officer of the Accident Centre at Frenchay Hospital as co-ordinator. The AEMT national training committee has since its conception included two qualified nurses with accident and emergency, intensive care or coronary care experience.

AEMT training, although primarily created for ambulance personnel, has now become more available than ever for nurses training in advanced skills and pre-hospital management (AEMT 1985). Its national training programme is based on four stages:

Stage 1 is concerned with anatomy and physiology. All systems are covered at a basic ambulance aid level and the respiratory, cardiovascular and nervous systems are taught to Registered General Nurse (RGN) standards.

Stage 2 concerns the treatment of medical and traumatic emergencies. All acute medical and surgical conditions are dealt with, including acute cardiac, nervous and respiratory conditions. A national examination can be taken at this point to allow, if satisfactory, continuation to stages three and four. A pass in the national examination also allows the student to become an associate member of the AEMT.

Stage 3 includes full patient assessment, practical resuscitation and ambulance aid.

Stage 4 covers in-hospital teaching in two parts: the action and understanding of emergency drugs and their legal restrictions, and in-service training within the Accident Department, Coronary Care Unit or theatres.

This part of the training enables students to undertake the practical skills of advanced life support: intubation, intravenous cannulation, recognition of cardiac arrhythmia and defibrillation.

The student must be found competent to perform 25 unassisted intubations and 25 cannulations. If found successful in all in-hospital practice and the final assessment of an external instructor, the student can be registered as an Emergency Medical Technician, AEMT.

It can be seen from the content of the AEMT course that many Accident and Emergency nurses would benefit from undertaking the course. Nurses would be able to use the anatomy and physiology instruction to update their own knowledge, and an organized study class would enhance their theoretical and practical skills in the care of acutely injured or ill patients in the initial period.

The National Staffs Committee training for ambulance personnel in advanced procedures is very similar to the AEMT course. Since the training is aimed to RGN standards, it seems reasonable that nurses should become involved in this course, which in a few years will become standard throughout the country.

4.9 AEROMEDICAL TRANSPORT

A different but very important form of pre-hospital care is required for patients who have been injured or taken ill while on holiday abroad.

With the increase in holidays abroad, the problem of transporting injured people back into the country has been a major problem. Many companies and organizations have seen the need to provide expert nursing and medical care continuing from the country of vacation to the home town. Patients may require intensive nursing while undertaking the journey and the nurses involved need to be skilled in this type of care.

St. John Aeromedical provides an extensive service with many nurses and doctors on call to help return a patient under their care. A patient with acute psychiatric illness can be returned with a trained psychiatric nurse in attendance, while patients with multiple injuries can have an experienced Accident and Emergency or Intensive Care nurse to care for their needs during transfer.

Care during the transport of such patients is not unlike the pre-hospital care required by victims of road traffic accidents. The one major difference is that often the acute care has already been provided to the returning patient, and what is required is expert nursing skills to continue the recovery.

This equipment, like that of a mobile emergency care team, must be compact and easily accessible. Most companies organizing transport for ill or injured people provide small holdalls and boxes to carry the necessary items. Unlike the mobile team, the nurse must not forget such items for nursing care as washing and toiletry arrangements. When called the nurse must be prepared with suitable clothing, equipment and an up-to-date knowledge of in-flight physiology.

Patients who may have need of advanced life support skills during the journey should be nursed by a person competent in this field of care. A monitor and defibrillator should be available on all flights on which patients suffering cardiac related disorders are travelling, and the nurse should be familiar with basic life support measures such as external cardiac massage and ventilation.

The Accident and Emergency nurse who participates in pre-hospital care is an ideal person for this type of work.

EDITOR'S NOTES

In this country and in others, A and E Departments' experiences of pre-hospital care vary considerably. In the US, pre-hospital care is a well-established part of the total care of the patient, but in the UK it is only just becoming established. Some of the difficulty stems from the question of who delivers the care, and, of course, the cost. Whether nurses, ambulance or fire personnel deliver the care, we must be clearly aware of what this care is, how it is provided, and the implications in our continuing care in the hospital.

Because of the diversity of experience and services offered, Gary Jones begins with basics and brings us up-to-date with current trends.

I have included in the Further Reading list some references to help you examine latest trends in equipment and devices used in pre-hospital care. Further reading on the positive and negative aspects of helicopter air-ambulances are also included in this list. As we become more sophisticated in our pre-hospital care, or live in countries where long distances are travelled, this will become a central issue.

REFERENCES

Association of Emergency Medical Technicians (1985) *Training Manual.* Peterborough District Hospital, Cambridgeshire.

Caroline, N. (1979) *Emergency Care in the Streets.* Little, Brown and Co., Boston, Mass.

Easton, K. (1977) *Rescue Emergency Care.* Heinemann, London.

Harrill, R., and Mather, S. (1985) Training of ambulancemen in the United Kingdom. *Care of the Critically Ill,* I (4), 14–16.

FURTHER READING

Jacobs, L.M. and Bennett, B. (eds) (1986) Helicopter EMS *Emergency Care Quarterly,* 2, 3.

Jacobs, L.M. and Bennett, B. (eds) (1987) *Equipment and Devices,* 11, 4.

Kerr, H.D. (1986) Prehospital emergency services and health maintenance organisation. *Annals of Emergency Medicine,* 15, 6.

Lloyd, K. (1987) Mast. and IV infusion – do they help in pre-hospital trauma management? *Annals of Emergency Medicine,* 16, 5.

Selfridge, J. and Dean, A.K. (1985) Mobile intensive care nurse preceptorship: a competency-based format. *Journal of Emergency Nursing,* 11, 6.

Smith, J.P., and Bodai, B.I. (1985) Guidelines for discontinuing pre-hospital CPR in the emergency department. *Annals of Emergency Medicine,* 14, 11.

Stewart, R.D. (1985) Pre-hospital care of trauma. *Trauma,* 3.

5

Disaster — Experiences with Civil Disturbance in Belfast

Kate O'Hanlon

5.1 PLANNING FOR A MAJOR DISASTER

What is a disaster? A disaster has been defined as an accident with so many casualties as to require extraordinary mobilization of emergency services (Rutherford 1973). In a small, inadequately staffed Accident and Emergency Unit two or three patients from an accident may be a disaster, while large numbers of patients can be absorbed into the daily workload of a large, well-equipped unit with adequate staff.

A definition based on numbers may be useful for statistical purposes but to use such a definition would present problems. For example, small numbers of severely injured patients, all requiring immediate treatment in the theatre, would stretch the resources of any hospital. A large number of emotionally shocked patients should not overload a large Accident and Emergency Unit.

Who first declares a disaster? Ambulance control will receive a request from the police, fire service or general public for ambulances to go to an incident. Depending on the information received on the type of incident and probable number of casualties, they will despatch the appropriate number of ambulances and then inform the designated hospital. The first crew to arrive at the scene will radio information back to control and the hospital. Senior ambulance officers will establish a control centre at the scene and also have a liaison officer in the hospital. All other emergencies should be sent to other hospitals.

Each hospital, area health board or authority must have an up-to-date disaster plan. Every member of staff must be fully cognizant of his role and of hospital policies. After each incident there must be a full staff meeting to discuss behaviour and problems. All hospital staff such as porters, security and pharmacists are involved in a major disaster, not just those in medical, nursing and administration services. A large wall notice of duties must be displayed in each area in a prominent position at all times.

The disaster plan will be distributed to each ward, theatre and all departments of the hospital. It is no good leaving it in a drawer and never reading it until five minutes before the casualties arrive. There should be rehearsals every six months: full rehearsal with casualties arriving, and ward rehearsal to discharge or move patients. The emergency beds should be erected and prepared for patients awaiting transport to other hospitals. All disaster plans must be flexible as no one can foresee the number of casualties, their mode of arrival, or the type and severity of their injuries. All victims may be dead but brought to a hospital for mortuary facilities and relatives' identification, for example, in the case of an air crash. Disasters may occur at weekends or evenings, when the staff is depleted, or they may occur when the department is full of seriously ill patients. Staff may have difficulty getting to the hospital because of riots or blocked roads.

Depending on the incident, casualties may arrive in small or large numbers. Initially the Accident and Emergency staff can cope but help will have to be rapidly mobilized. The department must be quickly restored to normality.

An Accident and Emergency Department must always be ready for any emergency. To cope with a disaster, nurses must be competent to treat patients on a normal day. They must know where all equipment is stored and be fully experienced in its use. The disaster plan must be fully explained to all nurses and they must know what is expected of them in a disaster. They must learn to appreciate that if they are sent to work in a specific area, they must stay there because it is there that they are most needed. Staff work more efficiently, quickly and with less stress if they perform duties during a disaster as similar as possible to their work on a normal day.

In some Accident and Emergency Departments, staff wear distinguishing coloured belts for easy recognition by strangers. Other units use colours for different areas, for example red armbands for a major area, blue for minor areas.

5.2 HOSPITAL MANAGEMENT

What are the problems in hospital during a disaster and how does a good disaster plan overcome them? Some important considerations are:

- initial communication
- correct staffing levels in the Accident and Emergency Department
- appropriate specialists available, such as neurosurgeons
- available beds for disaster victims
- information: press releases, public relations
- supplies, pharmaceuticals etc.
- security
- secretaries
- radiology
- operating theatres
- relatives

5.2.1 Communications

There should be a control team consisting of medical, lay and nursing administrators, the Accident and Emergency consultant and Sister. They will each carry a paging bleep effective within a thirty-mile radius. If unavailable they will hand their pager to a deputy. When answering a disaster call, they by-pass the hospital switchboard and ring the disaster telephone in the Accident and Emergency consultant's office. Sometimes the first news of a disaster is received directly by the nursing staff in the Accident and Emergency Department from ambulance control or the police. If the information is received by anyone other than the switchboard operators, the operators must be informed immediately as they are the initiators of the disaster plan.

5.2.2 Correct staffing

During the hours from 9:00 a.m. to 5:00 p.m. there is no problem with insufficient staff. In the early stages of a disaster extra staff will be required in the Accident and Emergency Department because of the simultaneous arrival of large numbers of patients. Some time will elapse before these patients are transferred to wards or theatres; these units will then need the extra staff.

An up-to-date telephone list of Accident and Emergency staff is handed to the deputized secretary who will call in staff after consultation with nursing administration and the Accident and Emergency Sister. Nursing staff is obtained from the College of Nursing, nursing residences and the wards. Sometimes the problem is not too few but too many well-meaning staff members. The nurse in charge must decide what staff are required and deploy them according to their experience, tactfully refusing help if it is not required. Experienced junior Accident and Emergency staff are often inhibited when nursing administrators with no Accident and Emergency experience arrive to help, and senior nurses are often reluctant to seek advice from juniors.

The Accident and Emergency consultant will decide the number of doctors required and their deployment. After assessing the patients, she will call in neurosurgeons, thoracic surgeons or others as required.

5.2.3 Beds

The ward sister or charge nurse will fill out Proformata 1, 2, 3, listing patients suitable for transfer within the hospital, to other hospitals, or for discharge (Figure 5.1). Nursing administrators will collect this information, which must be quickly available, and with the medical administrator they will arrange these discharges and transfers. Taxis may be used for those patients who are discharged home. A hospital entrance other than the one nearest to the Accident and Emergency Department will be used.

An area will be set up and staffed by experienced nurses with emergency beds to accommodate patients awaiting transport to other hospitals, for example in the gymnasium in the Department of Physical Medicine. Disaster patients are not sent to special wards unless these are set up in an emergency. The first casualties will go to the admission unit, theatres or Intensive Care Unit. When the admission ward is full the surgical ward on emergency take-in at that time will transfer or discharge patients to make available 15–20 beds. If more beds are required, all other patients are transferred until this surgical ward is full of disaster patients. The same procedure is used in other surgical wards and if necessary, the medical wards are used.

PROFORMA 1

WARD .... TOTAL NO. OF BEDS .... PATIENTS .... EMPTY BEDS ....

PATIENTS FIT FOR DISCHARGE

DATE ....

NAME AND UNIT NO.	DIAGNOSIS	STRETCHER	SITTING OR WALKING

PROFORMA 2

WARD ....

PATIENTS FIT FOR TRANSFER TO ANOTHER HOSPITAL

DATE ....

NAME AND UNIT NO.	DIAGNOSIS	STRETCHER	SITTING OR WALKING

PROFORMA 3

PATIENTS TRANSFERRED WITHIN THE HOSPITAL

Transfers from Ward No. ....

DATE ....

NAME AND UNIT NO.	DIAGNOSIS	TRANSFERRED TO WARD NO.

Figure 5.1 Proformata listing patients suitable for discharge (a) or transfer (b), (c)

5.2.4 Information

The receptionists will go round each area and write details of patients' names and addresses on case notes. As many details as possible are obtained about the patients' condition. The top two copies remain with the patient while the rest are taken by the receptionist, entered in the daily register in red ink (for easy identification) and also on Proforma 4 (Figure 5.2). As the patients are treated and discharged, the top copy of the case notes is quickly collected and entered in the register and on Proforma 4. Doctors must write the condition of their patients on this copy.

Three photocopies are made of Proforma 4. For one or two days after a disaster, the form is updated by the Enquiry Office as the patient's condition changes. For six hours after a disaster all enquiries are referred to this office. A 24-hour administrative control

PROFORMA 4

ANALYSIS OF PATIENTS FROM DISASTER

DATE ....

A. & E. NO.	UNIT NO.	NAME	ADDRESS		Ward	6a.m.	12 Noon	6p.m.	12 Mid.

UNDER DATE AND TIME COLUMN CODIFY CONDITION: 1. Critical   2. Serious but not Critical   3. Fair

Figure 5.2 Proforma giving information about disaster patients

post is set up at the reception desk. Officers are allocated duties by the administrator. For example, a liaison officer is responsible for each area health board and authority. A log book is kept by the hospital administrator to record significant events throughout the incident. In a major disaster, an incident centre is set up outside the hospital, either at the headquarters of the health board or in another hospital, and all information is passed to the liaison officer.

The public relations officer will undertake all public relations work either by being present in the hospital or by using information passed to him. No media personnel are permitted in the unit. The police will set up an incident centre in their headquarters and all external enquiries will be answered by them. Information is given to relatives as quickly as possible by the hospital liaison officer at the reception desk. Doctors or an Accident and Emergency Sister will speak to all relatives of seriously injured or dead patients. Unidentified patients wear an armband with the hospital number and a letter from A to M. This is recorded on a blackboard in the resuscitation room and the letter is not used again until the patient is identified.

5.2.5 Supplies

Initially there should be no problem with insufficient supplies in a well-stocked Accident and Emergency Department. The staff from the sterile supply department can open stores and replenish or resterilize supplies as required. However, trolleys may have to be borrowed and an adequate team of porters is essential.

A pharmacist may be needed in the Accident and Emergency Department to assist with the dispensing, checking and replenishing of drugs. There will be many controlled drugs dispensed during a disaster but correct, normal procedure can be followed even under the worst pressure, and no errors should occur in recording.

5.2.6 Security

The safe, rapid evacuation of casualties to a prepared hospital is essential in a disaster. The approach roads must be kept clear and inside the hospital grounds there must be no obstructions to and around the Accident and Emergency Department. Media personnel must not be permitted near the unit as they can prevent good access. If staff require assistance getting to the hospital, arrangements may

PROFORMA 7

SISTER, ACCIDENT AND EMERGENCY DEPARTMENT

Rehearsal ....

Alert   ....

Disaster   ....

Disaster information received at .... hours ....DATE

by ....

Source Ambulance Control   ....

Other   ....

Site of Disaster ....

Type of Disaster ....

No. of ambulances sent out ....

Possible number of casualties ....

Deputed Secretary

Notice received at ....

by ....

Contacted: Sister, A. & E. Department   ....hours

Consultant, A. & E. Department   ....hours

District Administrative Medical Officer   ....hours

Units Administrator — R.V.H.   ....hours

Nursing Administration   ....hours

Figure 5.3 Proforma 7 for alert to control team

have to be made for taxis to bring them. Relatives will be directed to the appropriate areas and all unauthorized spectators must be asked to leave.

5.2.7 Secretaries

Upon notification of a disaster, the Accident and Emergency Sister will ask a secretary to use the emergency phone in the consultant's office and give her Proforma 7 (Figure 5.3). The switchboard operator will set off the control team's pager and they will use this telephone to respond. The team proceeds directly to the department without phoning in to say they are coming, as this would tie up vital lines.

The secretary will stay in the consultant's office until the medical administrator arrives. He will be in overall control of the situation and will use this office as his base. He may require the secretary's services. If disaster occurs when a secretary is not on duty, any capable person may then be deputized to undertake these duties.

5.2.8 Radiology

An up-to-date list of the radiographers' telephone numbers is kept in the department. The duty radiographer, acting on information received from the Accident and Emergency Sister, will call in a radiologist and radiographers as required.

5.2.9 Theatres

Staff are called in at the discretion of the senior nurse and anaesthetic rooms and theatres are prepared. All patient enquiries are referred to Accident and Emergency reception for the first six hours. Patients' valuables and clothing, which may go with the patient to theatre, are listed and stored according to hospital policy. Bullets or weapons are handed to the police and must be entered in the appropriate book. A duplicate copy of the entry is retained by the hospital an a signature is obtained. This is important as there may be future legal proceedings.

5.2.10 Relatives

If there is a large number of patients' relatives, they should be in a waiting area away from the action of the Accident and Emergency Department. Information must be quickly available for relatives, initially giving the name and condition of casualties. A liaison officer, social worker or voluntary workers can be responsible for this duty, as well as tea-making facilities and telephones.

Relatives of seriously injured or dead patients will be brought to an appropriate room in the Accident and Emergency Department where the Sister or doctor will speak to them. A telephone should be provided for their use which by-passes the switchboard. Identification of patients brought in dead will be required. Again, the Sister or doctor will accompany relatives. The mortuary attendant should be warned of relatives' arrival as sometimes the bodies are badly mutilated and she can prepare the deceased for them. The presence of a police officer may be required during the identification and it is advisable to ask one to accompany relatives to the mortuary. This prevents extra stress for relatives who otherwise may have to identify a body twice.

5.3 THE SISTER'S ROLE IN ACCIDENT AND EMERGENCY DEPARTMENTS AFTER A DISASTER

The Sister is responsible for appointing the deputized secretary, giving her Proforma 7 with written details and directing her to the emergency phone in the consultant's office. She will respond to the bleeps of the control team's pagers, contact the Accident and Emergency consultant and advise nursing administration of the incident. All Accident and Emergency doctors on duty will be notified, as will the Radiography Department, receptionists and laboratories. (The nursing administrator is responsible for notifying theatres, wards etc.)

The Sister will ask doctors to treat patients in the department expeditiously and will arrange to move less seriously ill patients away from the resuscitation area. Ill patients will go to wards to be examined by ward physicians. Meanwhile, she will prepare the resuscitation room, instruct nurses as to their stations and duties and ensure that all areas have experienced nurses in charge. Senior nurses must observe closely the inexperienced staff and learners to protect them from undue distress from the horrific injuries and bereaved relatives.

After each incident, a staff meeting should be called to evaluate the experience of the staff; here, even the most junior nurse should feel free to talk about her worries. This meeting will help to identify organizational problems while the recall of the incident is still fresh. It will also help to discharge feelings of stress.

More frequently perhaps, the senior nurses might admit to having some fears. A good team spirit must prevail at all times in the unit among doctors, nurses, porters, receptionists and all other workers so that when a disaster occurs all work efficiently together as a team.

5.4 ARRIVAL OF PATIENTS

The Sister will sort out patients on arrival, making quick, clinical assessments and directing patients to the appropriate areas, that is, to the resuscitation room, major and minor cubicles, the day ward and dressing rooms.

A large area is useful in which emotionally shocked patients can wait until a doctor is free to examine them. All patients must be registered according to normal procedures. An experienced nurse must be in charge of this area because a patient may come into the department weeping hysterically and have some injury not readily seen. A nurse must observe all these patients. If necessary the transport officer will arrange for these patients to go home after treatment. The social worker may be asked to help with crisis counselling or a nurse with these skills may be used.

When all the casualties have arrived, the Sister must oversee the department, making sure that all the patients are adequately treated and all nurses are usefully employed. The doctor's and Sister's roles will overlap in many ways as the doctor also has to supervise the patient's treatment.

The surgeon responsible for take-in will organize theatre priority. Many doctors and nurses will go directly to help in resuscitation or the major areas; as a result there may be too many helpers. They must be directed to where they are most needed, for example in minor treatment areas. Nurse administrators should ensure that nurses are relieved from duty at regular intervals to prevent fatigue, irritability and impaired judgement. A fresh, experienced staff must be available to take over the department.

5.5 RECEPTION OF CASUALTIES FROM ACCIDENTS INVOLVING RADIOACTIVE MATERIAL

Some provision should be made in an up-to-date disaster plan for the reception of patients from radioactive emergencies. The following is a basis for such a plan that depends on the availability of quick, expert advice and help, and the location of the hospital.

A decontamination area must be designated. There should be a store in the Accident and Emergency Department containing:

- protective clothing for staff
- covering for floor, road and trolleys
- warning signs
- ropes and other equipment for sealing off areas
- cleansing agents (water may be used)
- disposable instruments and bags
- skin pencil

The names and telephone numbers of medical physicists must be readily obtainable. A radiation monitor must be available in the event of the delayed arrival of the physicist. Ambulance control should notify the designated hospital of the arrival of a contaminated patient, and the crew will remain in the ambulance until the entrance and floors have been covered; only on the instructions of the physicist will they bring their patient into the department.

The resuscitation of a badly traumatized patient must take precedence over decontamination of the patient. The fewest possible number of staff will treat the patient and they will remain in the protected area. The physicist will monitor the patient's areas of contamination and mark them with a skin pencil. Contaminated areas that are already marked with a skin pencil should be covered with a bulky wound dressing. The patient may have to be moved to theatre before decontamination is complete. The physicist should accompany the patient to ensure that there is no fresh contamination of new areas.

After the patient leaves, all staff working in the decontamination area are monitored. Walls, trolleys, sinks and so on must also be monitored and swabbed until clean. It is the responsibility of the physicist to dispose of all cleansing lotion, soiled clothing and equipment.

5.6 PLANNING FOR A DISASTER ALERT

A disaster plan should also contain instructions for an alert, for example when an airplane is unable to land at an airport. A two-seater plane with landing difficulties could cause a disaster by crashing into the terminal building or a built-up area. Instructions for an alert are similar in most respects to those for a disaster. The relevant staff are asked to stand by but may choose to come into the hospital. When the alert is safely over all staff previously informed must be notified to stand down; otherwise, an alert may proceed to the disaster plan.

The response to a disaster is not limited solely to the hospital: the ambulance, police, fire services, medical teams and social services all have an important role to play. On occasion the armed forces may be involved. It is advisable for all those involved in disaster management to meet regularly, to have 'mock' exercises and to become acquainted with their colleagues in other fields.

EDITOR'S NOTES

It is difficult to gain experience in the management of disaster, as disasters are, fortunately, infrequent events for most people. Civil disturbances, riots, explosions, gunshot wounds and all the ramifications of years of turmoil in Belfast have given Kate O'Hanlon a wealth of experience.

Those of you who know Kate will recognize her real presence in this chapter. It is this experience and breadth of knowledge that have made her very much in demand internationally to share her experience. Whilst the writing is essentially about Belfast, there are lessons for us all about clarity and brevity in our protocols, so that we can read them often and incorporate them. The clear and explicit instructions are so necessary to put some order into chaos.

For those of you who want to explore other major disasters further references are included on radiation emergencies. This subject usually merits high media interest. There are, of course, many other hazards in the environment and details can be found about some of these in the Further Reading list at the end of the chapter.

Local environmental hazards must be known to your Emergency Department and definite plans made to deal with these. A visit to the hazard site by staff, and a meeting with on-site experts always makes this a much more meaningful teaching situation.

FURTHER READING

DeBoer, J. and Baille, T. W. (eds) (1980) *Disaster: Medical organisation.* Pergamon Press, London.

Niles, R., Rund, D., Keller, M. and Saunders, W.B. (1985) *Environmental emergencies*. Saunders, Philadelphia.

Rutherford, E. (1973) Experience in the Accident and Emergency Department of the Royal Victoria Hospital with patients from civil disturbances in Belfast 1969–1972. *Injury*, **4**(3), 189–99.

Savage, P.E.A. (1979) *Disasters — Hospital planning*. Pergamon Press, London.

Turbiak, T.W. (1986) Environmental emergencies. *Emergency Care Quarterly*, **2**, 2.

Whittlake, W.A. (1985) Radiation exposure. *Topics in Emergency Medicine*, **17**, 1.

Yates, D.W. and Redmond, A.D. (1979) *Lecture notes on accident and emergency medicine*. Blackwell Scientific Publications, Bristol.

Yode, E. (1985) Hazardous materials response system. *Topics in Emergency Medicine*, **7**, 1.

Burns

Faxon, N.W. (1943) Management of the coconut grove burns at the Massachusetts General Hospital: The problems of the administration. *Annals of Surgery*, **117**(6), 803–8.

Wood, C., ed. (1986) *Accident and Emergency Burns: Lessons from the Bradford Disaster*. Royal Society of Medicine, London.

Terrorism and aircraft disasters

Jacobs, L.M., Goody, M.M. and Sinclair, A. (1983) The role of the trauma centre in disaster management. *Journal of Trauma*, **23**(8), 697–707.

Mass gatherings

Ayres, J., Hignell, A.F. and Skone, O.F. Visit of Pope John Paul II to Cardiff 2 June 1982. *Public Health* (London), **97**, 190–6.

6

Triage — A Nursing Care System

Peter Blythin

6.1 A DEFINITION OF TRIAGE

Triage simply means to choose, to classify or to sort. An assessment of the patient's injury or illness is made by a trained nurse to determine a true priority of care. Triage will not only ensure that the critically ill or injured receive immediate attention but also that all other patients receive care appropriate to their needs.

The origin and pronunciation of triage are French, yet it has received international application through a rather haphazard development. Despite its relatively recent connection with the management of patients in the Accident and Emergency Department, triage has a long and varied history. As early as 1700, the word was reserved for the food and textile industries in maintaining some degree of quality control. Similar segregation methods under the general designation of triage were used in many different situations and in many different countries.

In a medical context, triage is thought to have originated with the process of sorting casualties on the battlefields of both World Wars and other major conflicts. Originally triage described a hospital or medical station rather than a selection process. The formal selection process was initially part of a negative or reverse-order priority-setting system. As part of this system only the most viable casualties would be given prompt treatment, since they would recover quickly with a minimum amount of attention and be fit enough to return to the front. There was little point attending to those casualties who would require a great deal of intervention and effort. The limited medical and nursing resources at this time would appear to have legitimized such an application of triage.

Regardless of this rather negative yet practical adoption of the triage concept, the true potential of the system was quickly realized and developed. The experience gained from the management of large numbers of casualties, together with the increases in health care provision undoubtedly helped precipitate the development of triage as we know it today.

From these early and primitive interpretations, triage systems for assessing, sorting and managing patients were developed within a military framework. Indeed, many of the basic theories of sorting casualties out for evacuation from the front were included in combat training. Triage most certainly improved the quality of care given to those injured as a consequence of war, but more significantly, it gave rise to the introduction of life-saving measures applied before evacuation to established hospitals. The concept therefore came under close scrutiny. Triage was keenly developed within the military services to become an acceptable and proven method of caring for mass casualties in an organized manner. Its acceptance by the armed forces provided triage with a great deal of credibility which served to enhance its employment by non-military agents. It was soon realized that triage had a positive contribution to make to patient care within the provision of any emergency service (Figure 6.1).

Military triage steadily developed a more formal approach through recognized processes of evaluation prior to treatment or evacuation. As a result triage is now a well-organized clinical component of any military response to an emergency situation. Methods, systems and data concerning triage are subjected to constant analysis from experience gained during hostilities and disasters.

Disaster response triage and military triage systems are to a large extent compatible in that evaluation and evacuation form the basis of the protocols used. Emphasis is placed on the availablility of local resources so that optimum use can be made of such facilities. In both disaster response and military triage, priority setting has to be completed as the demand for care often temporarily exceeds the resources available. Triage has proved and continues to prove its worth in mass casualty situations.

A system of triage based on sound education and research was developed within the emergency departments of the United States. Initially such systems were practised by medical staff. However, it

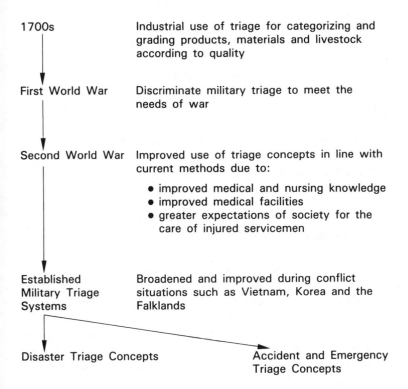

Figure 6.1 The Development of Triage

was quickly realized that an experienced and appropriately trained nurse could perform the triage role adequately. There is little doubt that doctors tired easily of this task and were more than happy to allow nurses to take their place. Since the early 1960s triage has become an important component of emergency room nursing in the United States and general texts and specific training manuals on it continue to appear.

Accident and Emergency triage has distinct and measurable similarities to both disaster and military triage systems. There can therefore be little doubt that Emergency Department triage has evolved from military concepts. All systems employ some initial sorting and priority setting. Nurses working in the Accident and Emergency Department have recognized the potential of using triage as an adjunct to planned patient care.

Given that planned patient care is designed to provide a framework within which nurses can give individual care to their patients whilst pursuing a particular model of nursing, triage must be seen as an essential prerequisite to this process. The purpose of Accident and Emergency triage is an initial evaluation of the nature and severity of each patient's complaint with a resultant plan of care based on the initial assessment. More individualized assessment is necessary as the nurse formulates a more elaborate plan of care responsive to each patient's needs. Triage assessment styles can be fashioned to whichever model of nursing is used.

6.2 HOW TRIAGE WORKS IN THE ACCIDENT AND EMERGENCY DEPARTMENT

Triage ensures immediate assessment of all patients arriving at the Accident and Emergency Department. It creates an environment conducive to high standards of patient care and management. The triage nurse, rather than a receptionist, is solely responsible for the screening of all patients arriving at the department. Switching this responsibility from a clerk to a trained nurse has advantages obvious to any nurse working in the Accident and Emergency Department as well as to the patients.

The main advantages of triage are:

- immediate or early patient assessment by a trained nurse of all patients arriving at the Accident and Emergency Department
- expedition of life-saving measures if required
- promotion of a safe environment for patient care in the waiting room
- provision of reliable information about those patients waiting for treatment
- effective screening of patients to establish true priorities of care
- early recognition of the needs of the patient's relatives and friends to identify those who require support and reassurance
- provision of the correct advice and First Aid when the patient checks into the department
- improved organization of patient care by utilizing resources effectively

- early and appropriate requests for case notes and X-rays
- improved public relations by providing initial and continued care for the waiting patients

To permit an efficient triage process, all patients must be assessed in a systematic manner which normally takes at most three to five minutes. This assessment takes account of the patient's appearance, vital signs, subjective and objective information about the illness or injury and results in a plan of care in the form of a primary clinical impression and priority rating. No assessment should be protracted; otherwise the process of triage would become counterproductive. Any critically ill patient is given immediate assistance and help is summoned. If a patient is expected because of prior warning from the ambulance service, the triage nurse will co-ordinate his or her arrival so that a delay at triage is avoided.

In addition to the formal triage assessment, the nurse will have to be vigilant in monitoring those patients awaiting triage when the system is busy. This may simply take the form of scanning the queue to identify the patient who may need to 'jump the queue'. This evaluation is not a formal process but may consist of checking for those patients who look sick or who appear anxious to receive attention.

Whilst the primary purpose of triage is to screen the patients and allocate a priority of care, the process also provides the opportunity to administer First Aid, give advice or implement any pertinent hospital policy. Requests for old casualty cards, case notes or X-rays can be made so that delays in securing such information are reduced significantly. Moreover, the doctor thereby has a greater chance of reviewing the information during his or her initial encounter with the patient and not after a lengthy delay that is often embarrassing, frustrating and unnecessary. If triage protocols permit the nurse to initiate the request for X-rays or investigations prior to medical consultation, then this should be organized as soon after the patient's arrival as possible.

Registration by the receptionist takes place once the triage decision has been made. Close communication and good working relationships between the triage area and the reception desk are important to the smooth running of the system. Completed triage documents are passed from triage to the receptionist either directly or by using the patient as a courier. The casualty card complete with triage notes to reveal priority ratings is then filed and should be accessible to the triage nurse and staff of the clinical area. Colour coding or a number system for identifying priority may be used.

Senior nursing and medical staff should be on hand to assist the triage nurse in the case of a difficult triage decision.

Supervision of those patients waiting for treatment ensures that changes in the patient's condition are more quickly observed. The waiting room becomes a 'known quantity'. Triage provides the nurse with details of all patients waiting for treatment so that when asked what the waiting room is like, the triage nurse will be able to give precise details of all patients, rather than just the number waiting.

Planned and spontaneous reassessment of the waiting patients enhances the reliability of the screening process by making sure that the initial assessment remains valid. Reassessments impress upon the patients that they have not been forgotten and that their waiting period is being given full consideration. No assessment is final and decisions may be changed in the light of additional information or a change in the patient's condition.

As part of the triage flow system, the nurse must ensure that the minor casualty or low priority patients are not left waiting for too long (Figure 6.2). The danger of any screening system is that it becomes advantageous to those who need care immediately but disadvantageous to those who do not need such care. The triage system must be designed so that this potential for error is recognized, and there is in the programme a means by which the triage nurse can filter low priority patients in order to keep the waiting times for this group in some sort of proportion. This is best achieved on a day-to-day basis through close liaison with the nurse in charge of the department.

Having made the primary assessment and established the priority for care, the nurse must assign the patient to the correct clinical area. This is of particular importance if the department is a large multi-function area with high patient turnover and throughput. Most departments have separate minor and major casualty treatment areas and may have other clinical areas such as dressing clinics, opthalmic treatment rooms, and so on. It is important to note that in the triage concept the waiting room must be considered as a clinical area of sorts. In addition to the usual sources of referral within the Accident and Emergency Department, the triage nurse may have other forms of referral at her disposal, depending on local policy and resources.

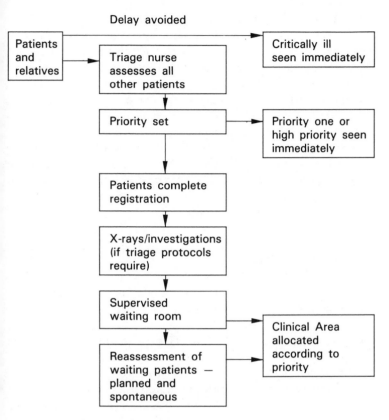

Figure 6.2   A Typical Triage Flow System

These may include:

- the nurse practitioner
- sexually transmitted disease clinic
- fracture clinic
- plaster room
- out-patient clinic
- social work department
- general practitioners
- community psychiatric nurses
- community nurses

The list is endless and is best constructed to meet local demand.

The active participation of the nurse practitioner in the Accident and Emergency Department will serve to enhance the role of the nurse in this speciality. The practitioner may act as the triage nurse or as a source of referral for the triage nurse. In this way many of the minor and trivial conditions can be dealt with quickly yet efficiently to the advantage of those patients who would have otherwise required the attention of a doctor.

The triage nurse has often been described as a 'traffic cop'. The description is apt for a major part of her or his function will be to control patient flow through the department and ensure that patients receive appropriate treatment. Triage will also provide a screening area for those only seeking information.

6.3 PATIENT ASSESSMENT

Immediate or early patient assessment by an appropriately experienced nurse is the most important goal of triage. Such a prompt assessment provides the patient and his family with expert attention at the point of check-in, thereby avoiding an unscreened and potentially harmful delay in the waiting room. Traditional practices have failed to offer the patient anything remotely resembling this. Notwithstanding the efficiency, effectiveness and experience of many casualty receptionists, the fact remains that patients are being triaged by unqualified staff. This practice, where it still exists, is totally undesirable and is tantamount to providing a second-rate service to the public.

In accepting that nurses are the most appropriate members of the team to perform triage, it becomes vital that they acquire the skills necessary to assess patients effectively. Assessment techniques involve much more than simply identifying an illness or injury correctly: the process must incorporate a wide range of activities related to nurse–patient interactions. Interpersonal skills may need to be developed more fully; indeed, they may need to be taught to enable nurses to function adequately as triage officers. Interview techniques will have to be refined to ensure that meaningful and appropriate responses are made during the triage encounter. Listening skills and the use of non-verbal and para-verbal behaviours should be explored in order to improve assessment techniques.

Nurses will have to document their examination of and interview with patients and their family or friends.

Documentation skills generally will require attention. The act of note-taking may be unfamiliar to nurses, yet it has to be mastered if triage is to be completed successfully. The nurse will need to be able to write a clear, concise and meaningful account of the patient's problems with a degree of speed. Clearly, there is little point in the triage nurse attempting to write the sort of notes more commonly found in ward kardex systems. Triage note-taking, for that is all it is, has to be straightforward if triage delays are to be avoided. Uncomplicated methods of triage records are the most successful.

It is important to realize that assessing and interviewing patients in the Accident and Emergency Department is not a new concept to nurses. Indeed, it is an integral part of the nurse's role. What is needed is for nurses to formalize this aspect of their work and recognize it as part of their role.

Whatever method of patient assessment is employed must be comprehensive yet brief enough to ensure the smooth and continuous functioning of the triage area and the department at large. Detailed assessments may be required for certain types of patients, particularly psychiatric patients or regular attenders for whom special consideration will have to be made. Such considerations may include the use of a back-up nurse for triage who could more comfortably deal with these kinds of patients.

The most common form of assessment in the Accident and Emergency Department is certainly the head-to-toe rapid visual survey with the elicitation of the patient's chief complaint. This form of nurse–patient interaction is all too often the basis upon which the nurse establishes a priority for treatment. Such superficial assessments can be dangerous and misleading, irrespective of how experienced the nurse might be. In making this statement I would not wish to underestimate the importance of experience and intuitive responses when making decisions about patients. It is most important that the value of experience is recognized but it must be used wisely when assessing patients. It is essential therefore that the nurse be competent at all aspects of screening so that the appropriate assessments are made and the appropriate decisions taken.

A common form of nursing assessment is that of a stage-by-stage approach to finding out about the patient and his family. This type of approach relies on information as the basis for making decisions

S = **S**ubjective information: what the patient tells you.

O = **O**bjective information: your findings on examination and interview.

A = **A**ssessment of all information: quick mental reference to all available information.

P = **P**lan of action: in the form of primary impressions, diagnosis and a priority of care.

E = **E**valuation: an ongoing evaluation of care whilst the patient is in the department. The nurse responsible for patient discharge or transfer can evaluate nursing interventions.

Figure 6.3 SOAPE Nursing Assessment

and is far more reliable and clinically sound than the visual survey described earlier. There can be little doubt that triage enables the nurse to apply such principles to patient care in the Accident and Emergency Department. The SOAPE format of primary evaluation outlined in Figure 6.3 provides the nurse with a definitive approach to patient assessment.

Subjective information is the evaluation of the patient's condition as the patient interprets it herself. Any pertinent past or current medical history, together with details of First Aid or pre-hospital care should be documented. It is important that the patient be given adequate opportunity to articulate her complaints and beliefs if the subjective evaluation is to be useful and reliable.

The objective evaluation should include assessment of general appearance, measurement of vital signs (where appropriate), examination of the site of injury and reference to behaviour if relevant. Examination of the patient must be simple and convenient with regard to the time and privacy available. This evaluation of measurable and observable detail can then be documented and compared with the subjective evaluation that the patient gave prior to making a decision.

6.4 PRIORITY SETTING

Priority setting is an important aspect of the triage concept and follows on logically from the nursing assessment. It is only through

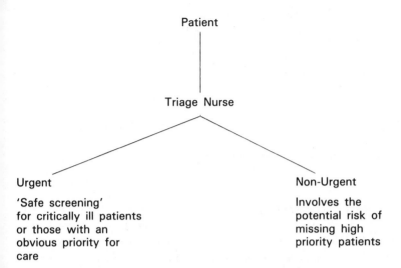

Figure 6.4 A Two-Category Priority-Setting System

a careful and thoughtful interpretation of the nursing assessment that an accurate priority for care can be applied to the patient. This urgency rating or categorization ensures that the patient receives the most appropriate care in light of the resources available and the demands being made on the service.

The triage nurse decides who will be seen by the doctor and when, depending on hospital policy. In making such a decision, the nurse must consider how long a delay the patient may be expected to tolerate safely. Urgency ratings ensure the establishment of true priorities of care based upon the acuteness or severity of the patient's condition. This screening primarily serves to expedite life-saving measures but also has the secondary effect of utilizing the resources available in the most effective way possible.

A reliable priority-setting system is the key to successful triage and may be interpreted in several ways. Whatever the interpretation, it fulfils the basic objective of classifying patients into two groups: those who need immediate attention and those who are able to wait for medical consultation (Figure 6.4). A system involving only two categories has often been described as a crude approach to triage that provides little in the way of meaningful screening. The danger exists

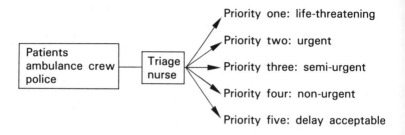

Figure 6.5 A Comprehensive Triage System

of making a generalized and inadequate assessment of the patient that fails to consider the situation properly. Despite these limitations, this form of triage screening may be sufficient to meet the demands of small Accident and Emergency Departments or minor casualty units in which waiting times and patient attendance figures are relatively low.

More detailed systems exemplify a commitment to meaningful priority setting and also allow planned reassessment of all patients with a high priority for care in the screening scheme. Reassessment may occur at frequent intervals, thereby avoiding the potential risk of deterioration and mismanagement whilst the patient is waiting. Figure 6.5 illustrates in general terms the form screening may take in a comprehensive triage programme.

Each hospital will have to decide the most effective and appropriate method of priority grouping in light of the resources available, department layout, patient flow patterns, patient attendance figures, local policy on treatments and interdepartmental relationships. Figure 6.6 illustrates a simpler and less comprehensive system of screening which is perhaps more easily managed. Whichever system a department decides to adopt or create must be based on the principle that all presenting patients have the right to an assessment prior to being allocated a priority rating.

Priority setting, however, can only be effective if it is organized within a more comprehensive system with full regard for nursing assessments. Many priorities for care in the Accident and Emergency Department are obvious. For example, the patient with central chest pain will be given priority over a patient with a sore throat. Many other obvious and simple examples demonstrate that traditional

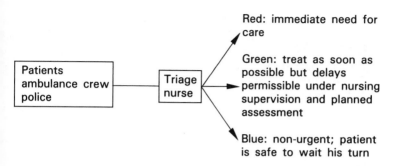

Figure 6.6 A Simplified Triage System

methods of screening in the Accident and Emergency Departments have always sought to safeguard the patient. But despite this rather comforting fact, there are many patients forced to wait longer than their condition permits because of inaccurate screening. A thorough examination and interview of patients with apparently minor injuries often reveals more pressing problems.

A comprehensive triage system permits the triage nurse to make adequate provision for every patient, be it immediate entry to the resuscitation room or simply taking a seat in the waiting room. Such triage programmes provide the nurse with a choice of several categories of priority into which the patient may be placed. The number and type of priorities designated is a decision that must be taken locally. Colour coding or numbering of priority designations is also a decision taken locally.

6.5 TRIAGE PROTOCOLS

The purpose of triage protocols is to standardize the response made to each patient, ensure that a safe response is made and provide reliable guidelines and a source of reference for the triage staff.

When deciding the format of the triage programme, it is necessary to include the use of triage protocols. Such protocols will need to be developed by both the medical and nursing staff in order to provide practical guidelines for the successful screening of patients. These protocols aim to standardize the response made to

Table 6.1   Care Priorities for Sample Injuries

Life-Threatening

  Multiple trauma
  Cardiac arrest
  Status asthmaticus

Urgent

  Severe haemorrhage
  Drug overdose
  Suicidal intentions

Semi-urgent

  Abdominal pain
  Fracture without complications
  Back pain

Non-urgent

  Rashes
  Local injury without complications
  Abscess

Delay Acceptable

  Social problems
  Constipation

Source: Compiled by the author

each patient with a given illness or injury whilst pursuing an individual approach to care through the nursing interview. The terms of reference established in the triage protocols must not inhibit the professional judgement or intuitive response of the nurse. The triage nurse should, through training and experience, be prepared to relate the protocol data to the individual each time a patient is assessed.

Triage protocols provide the less experienced nurse with a source of reference when the need arises. Standards of triage care can be set and maintained through careful planning of the protocols. In addition to these functions, such protocols serve well as an educational resource and training aid.

Triage protocols may take the form of notes, flow sheets, diagrammatic references or a standard documentation format. Whilst

Table 6.2 A Sample Triage Protocol for Lacerations

Subjective information

the site of injury
the time of injury
how injury happened
First Aid given
allergies
tetanus immunity status

Objective information

visual assessment
vital signs
location of wound
parameters of wound
depth of wound
type of bleeding
presence of FB
neurological status distal to wound
circulatory status distal to wound

Assessment and plan of care

Priority one	Priority two	Priority three
deep wound pulsatile bleeding; impaired circulatory or neurological status distal to wound shock presence of dangerous FB e.g. knife	heavy venous bleeding	minimal bleeding minimal injury

Plan	Plan	Plan
move patient to clinical area without delay	dress wound apply pressure elevate if possible reassess patient at planned intervals reassure patient while waiting	dress wound reassure patient while waiting

the provision of these protocols is important to the safe and smooth running of any triage programme, the triage nurse must always have access to a senior nursing colleague or doctor for advice when a decision is difficult to make.

Table 6.2 illustrates a simple triage protocol for lacerations.

6.6 DOCUMENTATION

Documentation of the triage nursing assessment is best organized as part of the casualty card. This permits continuity of note-taking, meaningful lines of communication, permanent storage of information and also prevents duplication of data. Should local medical and nursing policies not permit nurses writing on casualty cards, separate but compatible documents should be designed to meet the needs of the triage assessment. The use of separate documents for nursing assessments is fraught with the difficulties of keeping all the details about the patient together and should be considered fully before implementation.

The triage assessment may be recorded in detailed note form. This may prove impractical, but should not be excluded if it meets the needs of the desired system. Triage assessment records most commonly take the form of brief notes with standard abbreviations. Abbreviations and symbols for use within a system will have to be agreed and registered so as to prevent errors of interpretation. Preset information sheets, complete with appropriate memory aids and space for brief note-taking, are also widely used. Whichever system is adopted must ensure that the presentation of information is concise, clear and easily identified as the triage assessment. All triage notes should be signed by the assessing nurse and the time of assessment should be given.

Several attempts have been made to incorporate the triage assessment with the more elaborate write-up required in in-patient care plans. This is best achieved if the triage notes are used as a starting point or indicator for further areas of discussion and not as prescriptive treatment for the patient. No matter whether a planned patient care approach is intended for use in the department, the triage notes should form the basis of further note-taking in the clinical area. Triage notes start the process of nursing notes in the Accident and Emergency Department. It is entirely up to the individual department

Arrival in department	Planned reassessment every
	☐ 15 mins ☐ 30 mins ☐ Hour
Time triaged	
Subjective triage data	Objective triage data

Pertinent past history	Vital signs
	B/P Neuro. Obs. Chart ☐
	Temp. (Attached to Triage Form)
	Resp.
	Pulse

Relatives/friends

☐ Accompanying
☐ Following on
☐ Aware patient here
☐ Does not wish
   relatives to be
   informed

First aid at triage

☐ Dressing   ☐ Limb elevated
☐ Slings   ☐ Ice
☐ Rings   ☐ Splint
   removed

Other ....

Priority

Urgent   ☐
Semi-urgent ☐
Delay acceptable ☐

Notes (including reassessment notes)

Police involved
   Yes ☐ No ☐

P.C. Number.................

Station   ....

Signature of Triage Nurse

....

Figure 6.7 A Triage Form–Casualty Card

AGENT: ANIMAL .... HUMAN .... INSECT ....

LOCATION: ....

HOW LONG AGO? ....

FIRST AID GIVEN: ....

RESPONSE: ....

ASSOCIATED Sx: SKIN BROKEN .... BLEEDING .... SWELLING .... PAIN

RED STREAKING .... AREA WARM OR ERYTHEMATOUS ....

LIMITATION OF MOTION .... RESPIRATORY DISTRESS ....

PERTINENT PAST
HISTORY (IF ANY): .... TETANUS IMMUNITY STATUS ....

.... DRUG ALLERGIES ....

COMMENTS: ....

TIME: ....

SIGNED: ....

Figure 6.8 Triage Form for Bites

exactly how much is written about the patients, but I would stress the importance of documenting care, however briefly.

Figure 6.7 illustrates a triage form incorporated into the casualty card.

Figure 6.8 illustrates a triage form that has been specifically designed for a certain type of illness or injury. These forms are fairly standardized and offer direction to the triage nurse as to what questions should be asked and what should be looked for. The completed form accompanies the patient's casualty card.

6.7 TRIAGE AREA DESIGN

To permit efficient and purposeful screening of patients the triage area must be well placed so as to receive all arriving patients and maintain close contact with clerical staff at the reception area. Triage nurses are expected to liaise closely with staff of the clinical areas whilst supervising the waiting room. Although this may be difficult to achieve in practice, the concept must be accepted if the optimum benefits of triage are to be realized.

It is of vital importance that the triage area be equipped with a telephone and intercom or other such communication aids. Direct links with the ambulance service are also important in allowing the triage nurse to fulfil his commitment to co-ordinating the arrival of critically ill patients. A nurse-to-nurse emergency call system should be included with the communication equipment to provide a quick and relatively easy way of summoning help.

There is a need to strike a balance between the desire for patient privacy and the practical requirements of running a triage area. Confidentiality has to be preserved and is best achieved when some form of segregation between the waiting room and queue of patients is achieved. The use of private rooms can be counterproductive to the aims of the system because all patients should be observed whilst waiting. One method of gaining some level of patient privacy whilst maintaining contact with the waiting room is to construct a counter of sufficient height for the nurse to see over when standing but which ensures privacy when sitting down to talk to the patient. The problem with this form of triage area is that when intimate problems are to be discussed or a part of the body exposed for examination such as the breast, the patient should be attended in a private area in the main part of the department. Purpose-built triage areas will include provisions for all types of patient assessment and the use of private rooms. Whilst it is ideal to have a purpose-built area, triage can be carried out using a desk in the waiting room and the commitment of enthusiastic staff.

The triage area should be equipped with basic dressings and bandages to facilitate the application of First Aid.

6.8 INFECTION CONTROL

Infection control is an important objective of triage. Control should be instigated at the point of entry to the department and not after a period of suspicion during which precautions were not taken. The triage nurse will be able to alert the nurses of the clinical area of a problem and initiate any isolation or infection control policy.

The problem may be as simple as a child with measles presenting who has sustained a head injury. The triage nurse can transfer the child to an appropriate area and alert the staff of the need to observe the necessary precautions (Figure 6.9). The child's management is appropriate to her needs and those of the staff and patients in the department. More serious problems, if recognized, may require the involvement of the Infection Control nurse who would prove an asset to the patient's management.

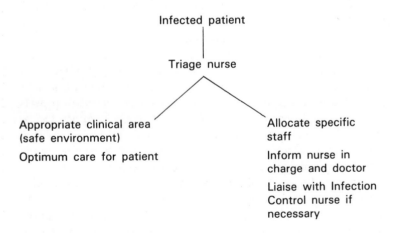

Figure 6.9 Infection Control Triage Procedure

6.9 PUBLIC RELATIONS

Immediate or early contact with a nurse at the point of entry into the department has the effect of reassuring the patient and his family. It inspires a degree of confidence in the service that is being offered and promotes rapport through this immediate interest in the patient's problems and the concerns of his relatives. Such a demonstration of concern enables the triage nurse to pursue a meaningful line of communication with the patient and his family, setting the tone for the patient's management throughout his stay in the department. First impressions count and there is no second chance to create a good impression. It is therefore important that the patient's encounter with the triage nurse be positive and mutually satisfying.

The patient and his family or friends may display anxiety, annoyance, aggression or impatience when asked to wait for treatment. If triage has been explained with the reassurance that assessment is an ongoing process, must of this understandable yet undesirable behaviour can be minimized. Information about the department and particularly about triage can be displayed in all public areas to aid patient education. Another successful form of communicating with the patient is to issue him with an information leaflet about the triage process following his assessment and priority setting.

Early and direct contact between the public and the nursing staff enables the triage nurse to assess the patient's relatives and friends and identify those who will require support and guidance. The triage nurse can offer advice with regard to what is likely to happen to their relatives and also keep them informed of what is currently happening. The flow of information to the waiting room is an important way to maintain good public relations.

6.10 IMPLEMENTATION AND PLANNING OF TRIAGE

Many factors must be considered in order to develop and implement triage successfully. The most important aspect of implementation is that the triage system has to be tailored to the requirements of the department and cannot be transposed directly from a textbook or triage manual. The idiosyncrasies, local policies, resources and location of each department all have to be considered with full regard for the principles of the triage concept. Each department has to design its own triage programme to meet the needs of the service.

When developing a triage programme, adequate preparation of both staff and the department are essential to its success. Initially all that may be required is that the topic be aired and discussed although it is vital that misinformation is avoided to prevent unfounded prejudice. A multidisciplinary approach should be fostered right from the start so that everybody feels involved and consulted. A working party to discuss the potential of the system and the management of change should be established. The principles here are straightforward and seek to disseminate accurate information about triage, involve all appropriate staff, stimulate debate and suggestion, and set the scene for change and development. Nursing staff will have to be prepared for their role. Time should be spent to ensure that a meaningful comprehension of triage is achieved and that the philosophy of planned patient care is fully appreciated. Opportunities for reviewing the available literature must be made for the nursing staff. Key and senior nurses should be appointed as educational facilitators capable of offering advice and guidance. In addition to the appreciation of triage concepts, nursing staff will have to establish acceptable levels of performance in many areas of their work. The following are important areas for which further training may be necessary:

- comprehension of triage to include the philosophy of planned patient care
- communication skills:
    - intraprofessional
    - interprofessional
    - nurse/patient/relative
- interview techniques
- observation skills
- documentation skills
- a comprehension of the United Kingdom Central Council's Code of Professional Conduct

This area of education is vast and will involve an ongoing learning process.

Triage protocols have to be written and tested. Medical and nursing staff must work closely together to secure satisfactory protocols that are both realistic and relevant to the goals of the system as a whole. They need to be easily read, accessible and constantly reviewed. Planned review dates must be stipulated to ensure that only the most appropriate and safest guidelines are used.

Public education will have to be addressed if triage is to be welcomed. The Community Health Council will aid this process of education and will be most keen to give its opinion of any innovation designed to improve patient care.

Once the concept of triage has been disseminated across the spectrum of interested parties, care should be taken to formulate a revised triage programme in light of comments from those consulted. This will appear as a fair process of consultation and offer a greater chance of success to the triage system.

Perhaps the greatest challenge to the implementation of triage is in seeking the support and approval of senior nurse managers and ultimately the health authority. The only way in which this can be met is by preparing a sound and well-documented statement of intent that illustrates clearly the unequivocal benefits for patients attending the Accident and Emergency Department.

Implementation takes time and should not be rushed. Careful planning and consultation should take place throughout the process of change. A pilot study to test each stage in the development of the new system is a reliable way of monitoring the progress and problems of implementation. Always be prepared to modify and change the original plans in order to achieve a system that is both acceptable and practical.

6.11 CONCLUSION

Triage is essential if Accident and Emergency nursing is to be practised well. The concept of early patient assessment before setting a priority for care is appropriate to the needs of all patients. Triage acknowledges the principles of planned patient care and begins a process that is logical and systematic in its approach to nursing in the Accident and Emergency Department.

Through triage, standards of care can be set, monitored and evaluated. The benefits to the patient are obvious and can be developed to ensure that only optimum service is given.

EDITOR'S NOTES

The work of the triage nurse is very stressful and is usually done under universal scrutiny. Decisions will need to be made under all sorts of pressure and the nurse's judgement will be evaluated. Insights, skills and structures to improve job satisfaction and other aspects of this nurse's role are particularly valued by emergency nurses.

What Peter Blythin does not tell you in his chapter is that he has considerable experience and expertise in this subject. He has studied triage not only in the UK but also in the US and Australia. His comprehensive bibliography I cannot add to, except for a reference to rapid decision making.

REFERENCES

Budassi, S.A., and Barber, J.M. (1985) *Emergency Nursing*. Mosby, Missouri.

Cormack, D.F.S. (1980) The nursing process: an application of the SOAPE model. *Nursing Times*, **52**, (4).

Kagan, C. (1987) *Interpersonal Skills in Nursing*. Croom Helm, London.

Kagan, C., Evans, J., and Kay, B. (1986) *A Manual of Interpersonal Skills for Nurses – An Experiential Approach*. Lippincott Nursing Series, London.

Landon, B. (1979) *Nursing Skill Book. Giving Emergency Care Competently*. Intermedical Communicator, Horsham, Pennsylvania.

Milne, D. (1985) The more things change the more they stay the same. *Journal of Advanced Nursing*, **10**, 39–45.

O'Brien, D., Clinton, M., and Cruddale, H. (1986) *Managing and Mismanaging Change*. Newcastle-Upon-Tyne Polytechnic, Sunderland District Health Authority.

Open University (1987) *Systematic Approach to Nursing*. OU, Milton Keynes.

Rund, D.A., and Rausch, T.S. (1982) *Triage*. Mosby, Missouri.

Thompson, J., and Daine, J.E. (1984) *Comprehensive Triage*. Reston, New York.

FURTHER READING

Baumann, M. and Bourbonnais, F.F. (1984) *Rapid Decision Making in Crisis Situations*. McGraw-Hill, Ryerson.

7

The Paediatrics Liaison Nurse and the Emergency Department

Hilary Wareing

7.1 BACKGROUND

A British Paediatric Association Working Party report in April 1982 on Primary Child Health Care in Inner Cities concluded that there was evidence to suggest that children living within the inner city received less than optimum primary care. A consequence of this is a high rate of attendance at hospital Accident and Emergency Departments. This is of particular concern since there is often a failure to follow-up these children within the community and this lack of continuity of care contributes to delays and failures in the detection of children at risk from abuse, accidents within the home and inadequate parental care.

Amongst the recommendations made was the proposal that Accident and Emergency Departments should engage a Liaison Health Visitor attached to the department, whose responsibility would be to advise primary health care team colleagues of attendances by their patients or clients following:

1. Potentially serious problems such as child abuse or accidental poisoning.
2. Inappropriate attendances for minor problems that could have been adequately treated within the general practice. This might help general practitioners and patients:
(a) to identify frequent attenders who might well have more serious underlying problems requiring assistance and advice;

(b) to identify areas where reorganization of existing practices would be of benefit to the patients.

A preliminary examination of locally collected data suggested that children living within the inner city areas of Leeds Western Health District have approximately twice the rate of attendance to the local A and E as children living in other areas of the district. In May and June 1984 a total of 1 135 children aged between birth and 14 years attended the department following accidents. Three-quarters of these children were 'self-referred'. Of these 1 135 children, some 86.3% were discharged home with no arrangements made for follow-up by the hospital and no communication sent to the general practitioner advising of the child's attendance at hospital.

It was proposed that a Research Health Visitor be appointed for a one-year period to be based within the A and E. The responsibilities of the appointment included:

- liaison between the A and E and members of the primary health care team concerning individuals attending the department
- recording specific epidemiological data concerning attendances by children at the A and E with a view to identifying both specific topics and neighbourhoods where health education activities need to be improved
- recording data to identify the reasons for, and the extent of, any difficulties experienced by patients in obtaining appropriate care within the community

Some may find it strange that a Health Visitor, usually based in the community, should be appointed to work in an A and E. In this chapter I hope to show the important role a Health Visitor can play as part of the A and E team. The aims on which a Health Visitor bases her practice are:

- the search for health needs
- the promotion of health-enhancing activities
- stimulation of awareness of health needs
- influence on policies affecting health

7.2 LIAISON

When I began working in the A and E the registration of patients was completed manually. Unfortunately the details requested did not include a date of birth, and other details were often scant. Gradually the system has changed with the implementation of the Computer-Based Accident and Emergency Records Project (CAER) and some gentle persuasion from myself. I spent time with the staff explaining the importance of recording details accurately and as fully as possible when a child attends the department.

Each morning I print a list of children less than 13 years of age who have attended the department the previous day. This provides me with brief details of each attendance and helps me to identify my priorities.

I retrieve the attendance cards from the files to obtain more detailed information about the attendance. These cards are filed in various places depending on any follow-up; sometimes it takes hours or days to find a card.

The medical and nursing staff leave me messages if they are concerned about a child who has attended the department. Whenever possible, I then discuss the attendance with the member of staff. Similarly, if I am concerned after reading the details on a record, I will discuss the attendance with the staff who attended to the child. Attendances that cause concern are not only those that may indicate child abuse. Injuries that are or could be serious and that are preventable are also warnings. Some are alarming because of the lack of supervision of the child, others because of a dangerous home environment. It is important that the community staff are informed of these attendances as the child may still be in danger.

If a visit is needed by the Health Visitor or School Nurse, if it is important that the information is given immediately, or I wish to discuss the attendance, a telephone call is made to the relevant person. A liaison form is made out for other attendances, giving details of the visit (Figure 7.1).

I invite the community staff to contact me for further information and to offer information which is relevant if the child attends the department in the future. Liaison is a two-way process and can involve many agencies and departments (Figure 7.2).

I use an index system to record details of children whose attendances need to be monitored and on whose cases I have taken action following their attendance. There are many reasons to enter a child's details into the index, such as:

In confidence

Notification of attendance at Accident and Emergency
Department, Leeds General Infirmary

From: Liaison Health Visitor
      Tel. No.

To:

Name of Patient: <u>D O B</u>

Address:

General practitioner:

Date of attendance:

Reason for attendance:

Treatment given:

Follow-up:

If you would like any further information or have any relevant
information to offer, please contact me.

Signed: Date:

Figure 7.1 A Liaison Form

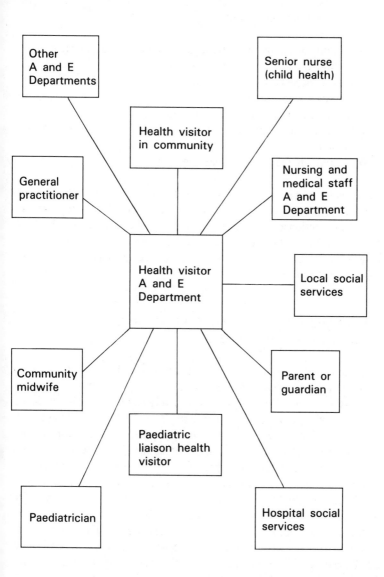

Figure 7.2 The Network of Health Visitor Liaisons

- a child or family who frequently attend the department
- a child on the Child Abuse Register
- where there is suspicion of child abuse or neglect
- parents who attend the department with overdoses or psychiatric problems that may affect the care of their child
- a child who has deliberately taken an overdose or harmed herself
- a child on the Missing Families List

Many have potentially serious problems such as accidental poisonings or frequent attendances for minor accidents and complaints. As has been mentioned earlier, the monitoring of attendances at hospital and follow-up in the community are important in the detection of children at risk from abuse, inadequate parental supervision, and a dangerous environment.

7.3 CHILDREN'S ATTENDANCES AT AN ACCIDENT AND EMERGENCY DEPARTMENT

Data collected over a six-month period about children of less than 13 years attending the Accident and Emergency Department at Leeds General Infirmary has shown that an average of 697 children under 13 years of age attended each month (Table 7.1). On average 363 of these children were less than five years old. These attendances accounted for 9.8% of all attendances at the department.

Data were collected for a period of one month to determine the sources of referral and method of departure. We found that 85.7% of children of less than five years were referred by the parents. Of all children under five who attended, 63.2% were sent home with no follow-up and 56.5% of these were referred by the parents. Of children five to fourteen years old, 85.4% were self-referred. After attendance, 61.9% of the children in this age group were sent home with no follow-up; 54.9% of these were self-referred.

The monitoring of attendances of children is a vital part of my work. At present when a child arrives at the A and E the reception staff do not automatically search for previous records. The nursing staff, medical staff or I must request the reception staff to search for previous records. We hope that in the near future the Computer-Based Accident and Emergency Records Project (CAER) will

Table 7.1 Log of Children's Arrival at the Accident and Emergency Department

	Mon.		Tues.		Wed.		Thurs.		Fri.		Sat.		Sun.	
	No.	%	No.	%	No.	%	No.	%	No.	%	No.	%	No.	%
Age: birth to 4 years														
1[a]	1	0.3	4	1.0	3	0.8	2	0.5	3	0.8	1	0.3	2	0.5
2[b]	35	8.9	28	7.1	26	6.6	19	4.8	18	4.6	39	9.9	50	12.7
3[c]	31	7.9	22	5.6	24	6.1	12	3.1	18	4.6	28	7.1	27	6.9
Age: 5 to 14 years														
1[a]	3	0.7	3	0.7	0	0.0	0	0.0	3	0.7	0	0.0	0	0.0
2[b]	37	8.5	29	6.6	33	7.6	32	7.3	32	7.3	30	6.9	43	9.8
3[c]	31	7.1	32	7.3	40	9.2	20	4.6	15	3.4	25	5.7	29	6.6

Source: Compiled by the author.

[a] Numeric pass band: 1–829

[b] Numeric pass band: 830–1700

[c] Numeric pass band: 1701–2400

provide a system to monitor the attendances of children of under five years, immediately alerting staff if a child has previously attended the department and giving brief details of the attendances.

7.4 CHILD ABUSE

Sometimes abuse is fairly obvious, but most of the time it is not. It is important that an accurate and detailed history is taken when a child presents at the A and E. If there is suspicion of abuse when the child is seen, a paediatrician is requested to see the child either in the department or in the Paediatric Unit. If I am on duty, I contact the Health Visitor, school nurse, senior nurse (child health) or Social Services Department to discover any relevant information about the family that may be of help in assessment of the situation.

Sometimes I become concerned when reading the record card

following the visit with the staff who treated the child. My concern may arise from the nature of the injury or complaint at this visit, previous visits by the child or family, details I know about the family or a combination of these factors. I always contact the Health Visitor and/or school nurse to discuss the details of the visit. The Social Services Department and the Paediatric Unit are also informed if the family is known to them. Depending on the results of the discussions the Child Abuse Procedure may be set in motion.

When medical or nursing staff are concerned about a child brought to the department during the evening, night or weekend when the Health Visitor is not available, they can contact the Emergency Social Worker and Paediatric Unit for advice and any relevant information they may have about the child. In some hospitals the names of children on the Child Abuse Register are available without the need to contact the Social Services Department.

Another way of helping staff in this situation is to devise a monitoring system. When a child has attended with an injury or complaint that has caused concern, the record card could be marked, thus alerting staff should the child attend in the future. A simple index system could be kept to give brief relevant details about the child such as the name of the attending social worker, health visitor or paediatrician. Any other important information should also be noted on this card. It is important, however, that staff realize that other children may be at risk in addition to those who are already known to be.

7.4.1 Recognition of signs of abuse

It is important to take particular care with children under two years (especially under one year) with fractures. A screaming, underweight infant or child may warrant admission or an early out-patient appointment. Be aware also of frequent attendances, which may indicate an underlying problem, a delay in seeking help or a discrepancy in the history of the injury. Other signs of possible abuse are injuries of different ages, a previous history of non-accidental injury and a generally distressed appearance and health of the child.

Child sexual abuse may present in many different ways: regressive behaviour such as a sudden onset of bed wetting, a disturbed sleep pattern, urinary infections, particularly in young children, discomfort or pain in the genital area or suicide attempts in older children. If in doubt as to whether a child has or has not been abused, a paediatric opinion should always be requested.

7.5 FREQUENT ATTENDERS

There are a number of children and families who regularly attend the A and E. Sometimes the injuries children attend with are in themselves worrying and they are referred to Social Services and/or the paediatricians. Such patients may attend with minor injuries or complaints and it is essential that agencies involved with the family are aware of the attendances as there may be an underlying problem. Other children attend with injuries that may not cause suspicion of abuse but are worrying because the child may be endangered by inadequate supervision or neglect.

Occasionally it is a parent who frequently attends the department. If it is determined that an adult who is attending frequently has children, immediate enquiries are made to ensure that the children are being cared for whilst the parent is in hospital and relevant agencies are informed of the attendances.

Travelling families often use the department instead of a general practitioner, whether or not they are registered with a practice. I try to build a rapport with these families and let them know where and when they can contact me. If there is a case conference or discussion about a travelling family who attends the department, I am invited to attend by Social Services so I can offer relevant information and gain information that may be relevant should the family attend the Department in the future.

7.6 SUDDEN INFANT DEATHS

One baby in every 500 live births dies suddenly and unexpectedly between the ages of one week and two years. There are about 2 000 of these deaths each year in the UK, accounting for half of all deaths in this age range.

During the last year, 12 babies between the ages of three weeks and six months who have died unexpectedly have been brought to the department where I am based. If I am available when the child arrives in the department, I stay with the parents while the medical and nursing staff are with the baby. At this time a brief history can be obtained, the other parent or relatives can be contacted and I can ensure that any other children are being cared for by a suitable person.

I remain with the parents after they have been informed that their child is dead. They are offered the opportunity to see and hold their baby and to return later if they wish to see their child again and perhaps bring grandparents. When the parents are ready to leave the department I offer to accompany them home and stay until family or friends arrive to give support. I give the family a copy of the leaflets *Information For Parents Following the Sudden and Unexpected Death of their Baby* and *What to do after a Death*. The former leaflet was prepared by the Foundation for the Study of Infant Deaths who have also prepared guidelines for A and E staff when an infant dies unexpectedly. I explain that the coroner's officer or a police officer will visit, reassuring them that this is routine following an unexpected death and that they are not being blamed for the death of their child.

The British Paediatric Association recommended that a single consultant paediatrician should co-ordinate a service in each district for families who have suffered a cot death. This development is under discussion in this health district and a consultant paediatrician with special interest has been nominated to develop the service.

7.7 SPECIAL NEEDS OF CHILDREN

Children should not be treated as adults. They have special needs of their own. The waiting area is important and anyone who has worked in an A and E knows what the main waiting area can be like, especially during evenings and weekends. Ideally there should be a separate waiting room or area for children and their parents. This should be suitably decorated and contain play material for a varying age range. In the department where I work the room is not ideal because of limited space. However, it provides a place in which children and parents can wait in comfort away from the main waiting area and with some distractions for the children. There are easy chairs, child-sized chairs, baby relaxers, a play table, blackboard, books and toys. The walls are decorated with a mural of Snow White and the Seven Dwarfs and pictures of nursery rhymes. This decorating theme should be continued in the room used for the child's treatment.

Children need a calm, unhurried atmosphere. When possible, the child should be treated by the same staff throughout his stay in the department. It is important when talking to a child to bend down to his level rather than standing in an upright position that may appear very threatening; it is also important to use language the child will understand. Some children dislike white coats and nurses' uniforms. This problem can easily be solved by the doctor discarding his coat and the nurse wearing a nursery apron.

Wherever possible, parents should be allowed to stay with their child during investigations and treatment. Parents need to be given information and support so that they can help their child and the staff.

7.8 HEALTH EDUCATION

The A and E is a place for treatment of injuries and complaints but it can also be a place for prevention education. Medical and nursing staff are in a position to influence future behaviour. They can provide advice and literature for parents that may prevent another accident. For example, when a child has scalded herself with water from a kettle by pulling the kettle lead or by pulling a pan off a cooker, the nurse can give advice about appropriate safety equipment and its availability.

The waiting area can be used to display accident prevention literature. Many health centres and clinics choose a different theme each month for their displays.

7.9 CONCLUSIONS

This chapter is based on experience and knowledge I have gained first as a Health Visitor working in an inner city area and more recently as a Health Visitor attached to an Accident and Emergency Department in the North East of England. I hope it has given an insight into the valuable role a Health Visitor can play as part of the nursing and medical team in an Accident and Emergency Department. The results of the research undertaken while I have been in post are now being prepared for publication and I hope those who have the opportunity of reading the reports will find them interesting and informative.

EDITOR'S NOTES

It was only when one of my children was hospitalized that I realized the amount of time and energy that is given by nurses to parents. The issues of children and illness, injury, abuse and death create strong feelings in both parents and staff.

This chapter addresses and emphasizes the importance of evaluating the child and his family in the context of the community in which he lives. It is so easy to make assumptions within the walls of the hospital and from the behaviour of parents and children under stress — assumptions that may be inaccurate.

In this chapter the interface and liaison between community and hospital are examined and given the attention they deserve. Often we have not had this valuable interchange, and many problems have ensued. The chapter also gives some insight into how the problems were highlighted and how the service was developed.

This makes the approach and ideas workable for us. It has much to teach us in our role in preventative medicine.

FURTHER READING

Bennet, B.R., and Jacobs, L.M. (1985) Accident prevention – health protection and promotion. *Emergency Care Quarterly*, **1**, 1.

Burton, L. (1975) *The Family Life of Sick Children*. Routledge and Kegan Paul, London.

Cahn, C. (1980) Care of the poisoned child. *Critical Care Quarterly*, **3**, 1.

Kelly, S.J. (1985) Interviewing the sexually abused child – principles and techniques. *Journal of Emergency Nursing*, **11**, 5.

McClain, M. (1985) Sudden infant death syndrome: an update. *Journal of Emergency Nursing*, **11**, 5.

Shockwiler, M.A. (1985) Parental stress after the unexpected admission of a child to the intensive care unit. *Critical Care Quarterly*, **8**, 1.

8

Sudden Death in the Emergency Department

Susan McGuinness

8.1 INTRODUCTION

Sudden death is always a devastating event. We need only a quick glance through the headlines of any daily newspaper to appreciate the tragedy and grief that a sudden bereavement can reap.

Every day, Accident and Emergency nurses are faced with the stressful and demanding role of caring for dying patients and spending time with their distressed and anxious relatives, accompanying these relatives on the first faltering steps of their bereavement journey through grief and their ultimate healthy adjustment to the loss of their loved one. Obviously such situations demand sensitive, informed and skillful management.

Caring for dying patients and suddenly bereaved relatives in the Accident and Emergency Department is an area that was for many years sadly neglected in the basic nurse training available to British nurses, including many well-qualified A and E nurses.

In general, newly appointed A and E nurses tend to look to their more senior nursing colleagues for leadership and guidance when they are confronted with sudden-death situations. However, this presents A and E nurses with a dilemma as many senior nurses believe they have learnt to care in these situations through experience or exposure to a large number of sudden deaths in the A and E. This I feel poses the question, 'Is "experience" of the kind I have described the best way, perhaps the only way one can learn how to care in such situations?' This question also presupposes that the A and E nurse has had an opportunity to reflect upon the experience and that the encounter has been a positive learning experience.

Many A and E nurses, myself included, still vividly remember after many years their first encounter with sudden death in the department. I believe that for some nurses these experiences, far from being helpful learning opportunities, have been experiences that the individual nurse would like to forget.

Obviously this is neither good management nor good practice. What then are the principles of care and guidelines that we need to incorporate into our management of sudden death situations in order to meet effectively the needs of the dying patient, suddenly bereaved relative and A and E nurses caring for them?

8.2 BRIEF SOCIOLOGICAL BACKGROUND TO DYING, DEATH AND BEREAVEMENT

Every A and E nurse belongs to a particular local community and larger society. We, like other members of that society, begin to form our attitudes to dying, death and bereavement from our early childhood experiences. These attitudes will be influenced by the family, local community and society in which we were raised and they will inevitably influence the care and understanding that we extend to dying patients, suddenly bereaved relatives and other members of the A and E team. The prevalent attitude within westernized society towards the denial of death has percolated through to the practice of modern medicine. Many lay people believe — and medical/nursing staff can perpetuate the myth — that modern medicine can cure all illness and save every life. Our perfected resuscitation techniques often serve to prolong the quantity of life at the expense of its quality.

Cartwright *et al.* (1973) stated:

A hundred years ago only 5% of deaths took place in hospitals and, even including workhouses and public lunatic asylums, the proportion was less than 10%. At the present time, the proportion is 60% and has been increasing steadily over the last twenty years. In urban areas, the proportion of hospital deaths is still higher at 70%.

Evidently this trend is increasing. Hedley Taylor (1984), reporting on the hospice movement in Britain, states: 'The care of the dying therefore is no longer the responsibility primarily of the "nearest and dearest'' but of white-coated doctors or rather uniformed nurses in Hospitals.'

In spite of the increased number of dying patients and suddenly bereaved relatives in the A and E, there is little evidence that the increase has been broadly acknowledged or allowed to influence the low priority many departments give to the training of their staff for this special responsibility. Only recently have A and E nurses begun to articulate research-based management guidelines and practice priorities for this specific situation.

The Centre for Policy on Ageing (1984), commenting on the changes that have taken place in society, stated:

The improvements in public health programmes during the 19th century allied to the decrease in child mortality during this century, have provided a state of affairs where larger numbers of people are living to a very old age and many of them, over a third, according to one survey, have outlived their relatives to care for them. At the same time the fall in the birth-rate following the First World War and the decreasing proportion of unmarried women since the Second World War has meant that there are fewer children – that is mainly daughters – to care for elderly parents, whilst the combination of job mobility and larger numbers of full-time working women, has had the effect of reducing the opportunity for caring on the part of those who do exist.

Equally important, the growth in medical science and technology since the 1930s, most of which has been concentrated in the large Hospital, has given the impression that only there is one assured of the best possible medical attention.

All of this has in turn produced a situation where death is an unfamiliar event, completely separate from everyday social settings, so that ordinary people have become increasingly less confident in dealing with it and hence reluctant to do so. In a busy, stressful and compartmentalised society it is simpler and safer to call in the medical (and nursing) experts to handle the situation.

These sociological developments have obvious consequences. Many adults, including A and E nurses, have never experienced a personal bereavement in their home or family and so they do not know how to handle it practically, emotionally or intellectually. The decline in the social rituals surrounding death and bereavement in society has resulted in the isolation of bereaved persons. They tend to be avoided by their friends and neighbours and so they are denied the opportunity to express openly their grief. Many bereaved people I have met have felt forsaken, misunderstood and unsupported by their family and friends during this painful and grief-stricken experience.

The lack of religious belief in an after-life denies many people in our society this small comfort in alleviating their grief and fear of death. Even though most A and E Departments are able to offer the suddenly bereaved the services of a hospital chaplain or appropriate religious minister, my experience is that for many relatives, God is irrelevant to the everyday events of their lives. Whilst relatives may very easily state their religious denomination, the A and E nurse has no information about the depth of their religious commitment, and the relatives' religious persuasion appears to provide many of them with little consolation at the time of their bereavement. Yet traditionally the hospital chaplain was the very person to whom we handed over the responsibility for the suddenly bereaved relatives.

There have been great advances in the development and utilization of various models of nursing care which have enabled nurses to decide their priorities in this area. However, the medical model still dominates conventional hospital practice. Thus we have a model geared to treating an illness itself rather than seeing a person with an illness.

In referring to the hospice movement, Sir George Young (1980) stated:

It is pointing to factors which have perhaps been forgotten in the medical profession's quest for cures and the nursing profession's striving for technical excellence. It reminds staff that there is an additional dimension to their patients; that we should not be so busy developing curative medicine that we forget to care for people as individuals where time in hospital is but a small part of their lives.

Hedley Taylor (1984) goes on to say:

Whether health professionals within the hospitals share this perception of their work — as concentrating on the complaint and losing sight of the individual — is another matter. Most doctors and nurses would claim that they too minister to the 'whole person'. Very few would actually subscribe to a 'medical model' which separates the symptoms of the illness from the patient experiencing them. Yet the experience of so many patients in hospital (and their relatives), however thankful and indebted to the specialist care received, suggests that, in spite of many exceptions, there is substance in these criticisms and that they apply with particular force to the situation of the dying.

These statements, I believe, challenge all A and E Departments to re-evaluate their care of dying patients and suddenly bereaved relatives.

8.3 EXPLORATORY PROJECTS

In 1983 the A and E team to which I belong decided to accept this challenge and to re-examine our management of sudden-death situations. At that time our management centred around the legal requirements and guidelines issued by the Department of Health and Social Security and our local health authority directives, such as informing the bereaved relatives of the involvement of the coroner.

As no training on the care of dying patients and suddenly bereaved relatives was provided for A and E staff by the local health authority, the type and quality of care available in the department fluctuated dramatically, depending on the expertise of the individual care-giver. This made it almost impossible to establish any baseline in the care we extended over and above the legal requirements mentioned above.

Unfortunately, despite an extensive literature search we found that little research had actually been carried out in this field, although a lot of material was available on the management of the terminally ill patient in ward areas or in their own home. There were no guidelines or principles of care in the management of sudden death in the A and E that we could readily adopt.

Therefore in 1983–84 I carried out two exploratory projects to try to remedy our situation.

8.3.1 First exploratory project

(a) *Introduction*

The aim of this project was to establish a national profile of the current range of care and facilities offered to the relatives of patients who died suddenly in the A and E.

(b) *Methods*

A structured questionnaire was devised containing 14 questions (see Appendix A). The questionnaire was distributed to 136 A and E Departments.

(c) *Composition of the sample*

The sample was selected from the *Accident and Emergency Yearbook* published by MMI (1982). Each department of the sample was listed as a 'Major Unit'. These had attendances ranging from 19 700 per year up to 109 893 per year (excluding Services Hospital, (6 505)). They were geographically distributed as follows:

England	104
Scotland	6
Wales	8
Northern Ireland	7
Ireland	8
Services (armed forces)	3
	—
	136

(d) *Response to the questionnaire*

The overall response to the questionnaire was very encouraging. The response rate was 98.5%, with only two hospitals declining to participate in the survey.

The findings are shown in Table 8.1. Many respondents were very frank in their comments:

Analysis of these replies may give the impression that we are uncaring when dealing with bereaved relatives. This is not so. One of our main complaints to management is our lack of space and privacy for patients and relatives.

Sister or trained staff try to spend as much time as possible with relatives. We talk about their deceased relatives, explain that everything possible that could have been done was done. Kindness and reassurance are the most essential factors.

Learner nurses do not accompany bereaved relatives now as they have been found to be overemotional.

1. Do you have a specific resuscitation area in your department?
85% Specific resuscitation area
5% Resuscitation area doubles as a theatre
5% A 'special room' but with no trolley
5% A 'special room' with trollies
(5% had a special room for the bodies of people 'dead-on-arrival'/'brought-in-dead')

2. How many patients can be treated in this specific area at any one time?
5% No trolley
45% 1 trolley
35% 2 trollies
15% 3 + trollies

3. Where do those accompanying the critically ill patient admitted to the resuscitation area wait after being separated from the patient on admission?
15% General waiting area
15% Sister's office
5% Doctor's office
45% Distressed relatives' room
20% Other: 5% Interview room
5% Chaplain's room
5% Treatment area/clinic room
5% Staff/coffee room

4. What facilities are available to accompanying friends/relatives of critically ill patients waiting in the department?
65% Access to public telephone
62% Access to private phone
35% No access to telephone in A and E
70% Access to vending machine in A and E 24 hours a day
5% Access to vending machine in A and E 8 hours a day
10% No facilities for refreshments in A and E
10% Nursing staff provide all refreshments
5% Tea is made in distressed relatives room

5. Do you contact the hospital chaplain?
Anglican   4% Always
                61% Sometimes
                28% Never
                 7% Only when requested
Roman Catholic 77% Always
                28% Sometimes
                 0% Never
                 2% Only when requested
Other   0% Always
                 3% Sometimes
                90% Never
                 0% Only when requested

6. Who usually tells the relatives/friends of the death?
20% Nurse
25% Doctor
55% Both
(Nurses only inform on the following occasions:
(a) language difficulties with overseas doctors;
(b) doctors' apprehension/reluctance to deliver news of the death;
(c) If the A and E nurse already knows the relatives.)

Table 8.1 (*cont'd*)

7. Do nurse learners accompany trained staff/doctors when caring for suddenly bereaved relatives?
0% Always
15% Frequently (unaccompanied by trained staff)
25% Frequently (supervised by trained staff)
5% Infrequently
55% Never, including occasions when:

(a) only pupil enrolled nurses are allocated to A and E

(b) nurse learners are encouraged to be interested but not involved in the care of suddenly bereaved relatives

(c) nurse learners are taught about care of patients and suddenly bereaved relatives in the school of nursing but they have no contact with suddenly bereaved relatives in the A and E

---

8. Do you give any literature to the relatives when they leave the department after a sudden death?
38% Yes
62% No

9. Do you only give verbal information to relatives about the implications (e.g. post-mortem)?
95% Yes
5% No

10. Who is responsible for looking after and liaising with the relatives when they are in the A and E?
2% Nursing officer
46% Senior Sister/Charge nurse
52% Trained member of nursing staff

---

11. How many of the following personnel usually come into contact with the relatives/friends for any length of time that suddenly bereaved relatives are in the A and E?
24% Nursing officer
91% Senior Sister/Charge nurse
92% Trained staff
62% Nurse learner
42% Nursing auxiliary
21% Domestic staff
63% Chaplain
25% Social worker
84% Police
66% Ambulance crew
33% Medical records officer
49% Coroner's officer
11% Nursing/General administration
2% Bereavement care Service

---

12. Is there any follow-up of relatives by the A and E once the relatives have left the department, e.g. telephoning them 24 hours after their bereavement?
7% Yes
93% No

---

13. Do you refer relatives for bereavement counselling?
10% Yes
90% No

---

14. Would you be interested in receiving any literature that may result from this research project regarding the care of bereaved relatives in the A and E?
95% Yes
5% No

(e) *Conclusions*

The most obvious impression gained from this survey was the wide variation in the range of facilities and type of care available to dying patients and suddenly bereaved relatives in the A and E Departments. I also discovered that my own department's situation was not unique and that other departments nation-wide found themselves with a similar dilemma. What appeared to be lacking were informed guidelines and principles of care specific to the management of sudden death which acknowledged that 'needs' in these situations were more than information on 'legal requirements'.

8.3.2 Second exploratory project

(a) *Introduction*

In an attempt to explore what these 'needs' might be, I carried out a second project over a period of one year, entitled 'The Nursing Management of Sudden Death in the Accident and Emergency Department' It was carried out in a busy A and E Department of a London teaching hospital.

(b) *Literature review*

I began my second project by carrying out a literature review. Briefly summarized, my objectives and conclusions were as follows:

(i) *To identify a general sociological background to loss, dying, death and bereavement.* Studies by Friedson (1961), Lessa and Vogt (1965), Elder (1973) and Rudy (1980) have shown that people generally strive to control their social and physical environment and to determine or at least strive to have prior knowledge of what happens in their own lives. This dynamic of seeking information in order to interpret and understand what is happening to ourselves is one I have met in many distressed and anxious relatives accompanying dying patients in A and E Departments. It underlines how important a role A and E staff play both in providing relatives with relevant and honest information at this time and in facilitating the relatives' understanding of this information. Distressed and anxious relatives must not simply be left in a confused state, sitting in a general waiting area or a distressed relatives room drinking cups of tea!

Studies by Hoffman (1978), Vachon *et al.* (1978), Parkes (1981) and Bowling (1983) indicate a significant development in our understanding of the relationship between different personality types and grief processes. This illustrates the point that we can only interpret and understand what is happening to us as unique individuals with our own personalities, reacting to a crisis situation often not as we would like to, but as the people that we are — perhaps silent, aggressive or hysterical.

(ii) To identify the needs of patients, relatives and the nursing staff in sudden death situations

1. Commenting on the needs of dying patients, a study by the Centre for Policy on Ageing (1983) suggested that although care may be given to the physical needs of dying patients in hospital, not enough time is given to the emotional, psychological, intellectual, spiritual and sociocultural needs of the patient.
2. In reviewing the needs of bereaved relatives, Gerber *et al.* (1975), Raphael (1977), Parkes (1980, 1981) and Le Poidevan (1983) emphasized a holistic approach to grief and mourning and an appreciation of the uniqueness of any individual's response to loss, particularly a bereavement.
3. Studies by Wright (1980), Forrest *et al.* (1982) and Thompson (1983) of the needs of nursing staff in facilitating a healthy adjustment to loss emphasized the need for nursing staff to be able to own and accept the emotional pain or lack of it. These authors explored the experience of spending time with those suffering a loss, which can arouse grief and mourning in the carer, particularly in sudden infant death situations. They also identified the need for non-judgemental support from the nursing team to facilitate the expression of these feelings and thereby provide a means for the healthy resolution of the emotional pain.

Studies by Wilson (1977), and Ainsworth-Smith and Speck (1982) identified the spiritual needs of dying patients, bereaved relatives and the nursing staff caring for them.

(iii) To establish practice guidelines recommended in previous studies in the adjustment to loss that are applicable to the nursing management of sudden death and bereavement in the A and E. The Oxford Study (Forrest *et al.* 1982) reviewed the practice guidelines drawn

up four years previously by the National Stillborn Study Group. These guidelines were aimed at facilitating the mourning of a stillborn baby, although the principles involved are, I feel, relevant to any sudden bereavement. These include seeing and holding the baby after the death, naming him or her, taking part in the funeral arrangements and being informed about the cause of the baby's death, future pregnancies and any genetic implications through discussion with nursing and medical staff.

The implementation and practice of these guidelines were found to have had an important contribution to the parents' adjustment to their bereavement. The report concluded:

There is a lot of evidence that there is widespread ignorance and misconception about how to help bereaved people, and there clearly needs to be much more education of the general public about these matters.

This statement could be applied not only to the general public but to the medical and nursing professions as a whole.

Parkes (1980) recommended that those caring for the bereaved should be trained in psychosocial skills. His study suggested that factual knowledge, although important, was not enough when communicating with and supporting distressed people. More importantly, the correct attitude and the development of communication skills are essential to ensure a healthy resolution of grief.

(c) *Methods*

In this study a combination of methods were used to accumulate data. These were:

1. Observation periods: I spent one day and night each week in the A and E observing a particular shift on-duty (Figure 8.1). The shift system in this A and E operates 24 hours a day, 7 days a week. The 24-hour day is divided into three shifts: 7:30 a.m. to 4:30 p.m., 1:00 p.m. to 9.30 p.m. and 9:30 p.m. to 7:30 a.m.
2. A structured questionnaire (Appendix B) was distributed to a cross-sectional sample of the nursing staff.
3. Follow-up interviews took place when the completed questionnaires were returned.

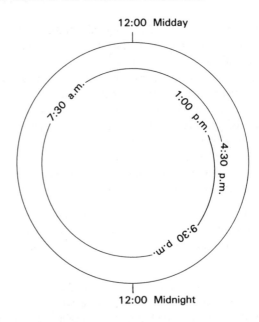

Figure 8.1 Shift Rotation in the Accident and Emergency Department

(d) *Distribution of questionnaire*

This questionnaire was distributed to a cross-sectional sample of the qualified nursing staff and nurse learners in the A and E. The sample of 17 included more than half the total complement of nursing staff/learners in the department during the period under survey.

(e) *Response to questionnaire*

From this sample of 17, 88.6% responded to the questionnaire, 75.8% completed it, and 12.8% completed both the questionnaire and the structured interview. Almost two-thirds of the sample (64.7%) requested a copy of the data analysis and the conclusions of the project.

(f) *Brief comments on analysis of data*

The respondents found dealing with sudden-death situations stressful. Evidence suggested that the more senior nurses were more confident and positive in their response to sudden-death situations, while junior nurses associated negative feelings and attitudes with dealing with sudden death and bereaved relatives. Why is this? Perhaps, as one senior nurse commented, 'I think one can't afford to let it affect you. I don't mean you're never affected at all but one becomes better at hiding it.'

It is undoubtedly important that in learning to cope with repeated situations of dying and bereavement, a nurse is not emotionally disabled and unable to function. Neither, however, should one be detached from one's honest feelings. Most importantly, dying patients and bereaved relatives should not feel inhibited from having a healthy, appropriate reaction to the death of their loved one.

Sadly, an awareness of the needs of suddenly bereaved relatives and the desire for A and E nurses to spend time creatively with them was not seen by senior nurses as a skill for which A and E nurses needed preparation and training to develop, or opportunities to reflect upon. In general, nurse learners and the qualified nursing staff appeared to be unaware of the availability of appropriate literature for bereaved relatives or the existence of a bereavement support group within the hospital.

The small amount of information given to nurses in the A and E about the management of sudden-death situations was criticized by one senior nurse participant, who presented this information to junior nursing staff. She described it as 'something slipped in, if you like, and they possibly think it's slipped in as well and that's deliberate so as not to make it too much of an issue.'

Interestingly, when asked whose responsibility it was to encourage the development of caring skills for the bereaved amongst A and E nurses, one senior nurse stated:

I see it as someone else's, quite whose I'm not sure. It's funny really, it becomes very difficult. We're hidebound with rules and then along comes an important subject and you say, 'Hard luck, do your own thing with this one.'

The respondents readily identified the educational requirements most necessary to supplement their existing 'example and experience' type of preparation. These fell into three categories:

1. The need to be more informed about the resources available in the local community, such as the role of the general practitioner and Social Services following a sudden death.

2. The opportunity to develop and improve communication skills, specifically dealing with dying patients and their families.
3. Opportunities for A and E nurses to share and discuss their experiences of dealing with sudden-death situations in group sessions. This would enable a supportive and learning dimension to be integrated into nurses' experience of A and E nursing.

Interestingly, categories 2 and 3 above were identified solely by the junior nursing staff in the sample.

My research project concluded with four recommendations:

1. To re-examine the current orientation programme for nurse learners and qualified staff in managing sudden-death situations, in the light of the research findings.
2. The implementation of a holistic person-centred model of care that meets the needs of dying patients, suddenly bereaved relatives and the nursing staff as identified in the report.
3. The provision of in-service training opportunities for all levels of nursing and medical staff to develop the essential communications skills needed in caring for the suddenly bereaved.
4. The provision of nursing supervision and support groups in which staff can air their feelings and attitudes towards sudden death and bereavement in the A and E.

8.4 GUIDELINES FOR THE MANAGEMENT OF SUDDEN-DEATH SITUATIONS IN THE A AND E

Since 1983, I have been employed as a full-time staff nurse/bereavement counsellor in the Accident and Emergency Department of Hope Hospital, Salford. We, as the Accident and Emergency team, were committed to allowing the practice guidelines, principles of care and research recommendations identified earlier in the literature review to inform our management of sudden-death situations in the A and E. Gradually over the last three years, we have implemented changes in our management of sudden death and we have endeavoured to strive for a more informed way of caring for dying patients and suddenly bereaved relatives. These include the relatives of those who are already 'dead on arrival' who can turn up unexpectedly in A and E Departments unaware that their loved one is dead.

The aim of our care of suddenly bereaved relatives is to facilitate their acceptance of the death and their adjustment to loss. Listed below are some practical measures that we have found useful.

8.4.1 Relatives' room

In our A and E we have a relatives' room to provide a comfortable and private environment for the relatives and friends of dying patients. It is pleasantly decorated and furnished, with a kettle and other facilities for making refreshments. We also keep our bereavement literature and other relevant information and telephone numbers in a cupboard in the room. There is a telephone and local telephone directories available for the relatives. The room is located near the reception desk, resuscitation area and toilets, providing easy access to these areas for distressed and grieving relatives who are often embarrassed and disorientated by their emotional reactions to the crisis in which they find themselves.

8.4.2 Reception

When relatives arrive in the department, if the nurse responsible for the care of the relatives is not immediately available, the A and E reception staff will have been informed as to his or her name and will page the particular nurse after accompanying the relatives to the relatives' room.

8.4.3 Resuscitation team liaison

It is essential that there is continuous liaison between the resuscitation team and the relatives of the dying patient. Care of the relatives is carried out by a designated nurse in the A and E. If I am on duty, I will 'be there' for the relatives whilst the resuscitation team stays with the patient. I have free access to the resuscitation area and can see how the resuscitation is progressing, consulting the senior doctor about its most likely outcome. This also gives me an opportunity to establish a rapport with the relatives and enables me to find out what the relatives know of the circumstances preceding the patient's admission to the A and E. If I am not on duty another nurse will follow the same approach with the relatives and 'be there' for them.

8.4.4 Notifying the relatives

In some instances no relatives accompany patients to the hospital and no next-of-kin is aware of the situation. In these instances we check our computer records for previous admissions of the patient in the hope that a name, address and telephone number may have been recorded of a relative/neighbour/warden/social worker whom we can contact.

If there is no previous record of admission, the nurse will examine the patient's clothing and property for clues as to the patient's identity and use agencies such as the general practitioner, police or council housing offices to contact relatives.

8.4.5 The roles of the chaplain and social worker

We liaise with other available services, such as the hospital chaplain or social worker. The patient or relatives may already be known to the chaplain and a familiar face at such a distressing time can be of great comfort to the family. The hospital chaplain may also provide relatives with help later in arranging a funeral. This is especially significant if the family does not belong to any particular local church community, a common situation in inner-city areas. The social worker may also provide help and advice for grants available to the family towards the cost of a funeral. The inability of a family to pay for a funeral can often be a very distressing factor in their subsequent grief.

Many families, especially those in which small babies or children have died suddenly, experience a great deal of guilt at being unable to provide a 'decent' burial. Unfortunately, with a high level of unemployment and an increase in the number of single-parent families, this is becoming a more common situation and the stigma of a 'pauper's grave' still flourishes.

8.4.6 Supporting the relatives

We also contact other relatives or friends if a relative is waiting alone in the A and E, and ask them to come to the department. Relatives may have to spend time after the death of the patient waiting for a coroner's officer to meet them in order to identify the deceased's body and a familiar face can often give the relative permission to begin to grieve.

If necessary we contact schools in order to alert them to the situation and to co-ordinate arrangements for children to be picked up from school.

8.4.7 Obtaining a medical history

We rely on the relative as an important source of information about the patient's previous medical history. This information can sometimes be invaluable to the resuscitation team. We have had occasions when a patient was thought to have a marvellous suntan from a Mediterranean holiday and in fact was terminally ill after a long period of chemotherapy. It is best to obtain this type of information as soon as possible as it can influence the resuscitation procedure and the relatives can become rapidly disorientated and confused as fear and anxiety overwhelm them during their time in the department.

8.4.8 Anticipatory grief work

Anticipatory grief work means preparing relatives for the most likely outcome of the resuscitation. All too often, in a distressing and tragic situation it is much easier for the nurse to be dishonest with relatives about the progress of the resuscitation and to give relatives false hope in a hopeless situation. When relatives ask how the patient is and if she is going to 'make it', it is easier for the nurse to avoid answering their questions and perhaps respond by saying, 'She is in the best place' or 'The doctors are doing their best'. It is more difficult but far better to be honest with relatives and say, 'Your husband is really very seriously ill and he has still not responded to any of the drugs we have given him'.

As the nurse observes the course of the resuscitation she may consult the senior doctor about its progress and perhaps have to tell the relatives that the person they know and love is dying. If the nurse has been honest with relatives and begun the anticipatory grief work, then she will have enabled them to be receptive to this information and in a sense, have begun the bereavement journey with the relatives, bringing them slowly to the awful realization that, far from being just a horrible nightmare, the events of the last few minutes or hours are really happening.

8.4.9 Accompanying the patient

We encourage the relatives to enter the resuscitation area to be with the person they know and love. They are usually accompanied by the chaplain to pray with and for the dying patient. This is important as it is all too easy for the A and E team to dispossess the families of the person they love. These are usually occasions in which the resuscitation has been discontinued or the person is terminally ill and obviously dying. This enables the relatives and friends to say their goodbyes and to be with the dying patient. Obviously, we prepare the relatives for the scene they will meet when they come into the resuscitation area and support them throughout this time. It also enables us to reinforce the reality of what is happening as many relatives may be in a state of shock and disbelief, perhaps even denial, because of the sudden and unexpected nature of the event.

8.4.10 Informing relatives of the patient's death

Relatives are usually informed of the patient's death by the trained member of staff they have come to know best, usually a nurse. The senior doctor at the resuscitation also comes to speak to the relatives and explains what is believed to have caused the death of the patient. They then try to answer the relatives' questions.

Our intention here is to listen to the relatives' reactions to the news of the death, to reinforce the information we want to communicate to the relatives and to accept their reactions, their personal response to this devastating tragedy. These reactions can include great periods of silence, guilt, physical or verbal violence, sometimes misdirected towards the nursing and medical staff.

There are no easy ways of breaking bad news to a suddenly bereaved relative but we try to be aware of a few basic principles. These include:

- spending a few moments preparing oneself for the task in hand
- thinking about how and what you are going to say to the relatives
- building on previous information given to the relatives (see point 8) through the anticipatory grief work
- trying to avoid cliches and jargon such as, 'I'm afraid we've lost him'. These are unhelpful for relatives, who are already confused, afraid and disorientated by the events of the day

- taking your time breaking bad news, giving yourself two or three sentences as a lead-in to the actual news of the death of the patient
- choosing appropriate vocabulary, talking neither up nor down to the relatives, but meeting the relatives where they are.

8.4.11 Viewing the body of the deceased

We encourage relatives to view the body of the deceased person. If the relatives arrive after the patient has died and the relatives wish, the hospital chaplain may accompany the relatives to view the body and pray for the deceased patient. This provides the relatives with an opportunity to say their goodbyes. If the deceased patient is a child or baby, we encourage the parents to hold the baby or child in their arms, and we offer the possibility of an instant photograph of the baby to the parents.

Very often parents will have many photographs of the baby at the time of his or her birth. What tends to happen is that they do not have any photographs of the baby between three and nine months, when the baby looks very different. Parents after they have experienced Sudden Infant Death Syndrome often agonize over the fact that only a few months after their baby's death they are unable to remember what he or she looked like and the photograph can provide a focus for their grief. Some parents decline the immediate offer of a photograph and I file these photographs for one year, as my experience is that sometimes parents may ask for the photograph much later in their bereavement.

8.4.12 Immediate care for the relatives

Once the news of the death has been communicated to the relatives we try to spend time simply 'being with' them rather than 'doing for' them. The amount of time varies from relative to relative and the particular circumstances of the death.

We explain the legal implications of a sudden death, such as involvement of the coroner's office and officers. We have a good working relationship with these two officers, who are very caring, supportive and helpful towards the relatives.

We provide literature for relatives explaining the factual information they need to know about the legal implications of a death of a loved one. This includes leaflets from the Department of Health and Social Security (*What to do after a death* and *Death Grant*) and the Welfare Right's Office (*Funeral Costs*). We are currently rewriting, as an accompaniment to the Department of Health and Social Security literature, an explanation of the ways that grief can express itself.

We try to ensure that the relatives have transport home and try to arrange for a relative or friend to spend the night with the bereaved person.

8.4.13 Follow-up care for the relatives

We try to obtain a telephone number at which relatives can be contacted in the next few days, so that the staff nurse bereavement counsellor can contact them. This gives the relatives the opportunity to ask any questions they may have surrounding the death and also offers the A and E staff the opportunity of expressing their concern.

We also try to contact the GP, Health Visitor, and so on, to alert them to the fact of the death. We offer all 'cot-death' parents the opportunity of immediate support from the local cot-death support group which is comprised of other parents who have experienced cot-deaths. They are available 24 hours a day, seven days a week.

8.4.14 In the weeks ahead

As the staff nurse bereavement counsellor, I am available to the relatives for short-term bereavement counselling. My experience is that the majority of suddenly bereaved relatives do not need bereavement counselling, but some relatives do. These relatives tend to be isolated with no obvious social support in the form of family or friends. This is a particularly common situation, for example, with older married couples who have had no children and who have spent their lives devoted to each other and where a husband or wife dies suddenly. Suddenly bereaved relatives whom other A and E nursing staff have cared for and about whom they are concerned are referred to me by my colleague for a follow-up visit.

At a later date, usually a week or two later, I contact the relatives and if they wish I visit them in their own home. Some relatives will need just the one visit but to others I offer the opportunity of short-term bereavement counselling.

The counselling model I use is Le Poidevan's Model of Adjustment to Loss and Change (Appendix C).

8.4.15 What about the A and E team?

It is obviously stressful for nursing and medical staff to be constantly confronted with tragic situations. We are attempting to establish a support group for trained staff in high-dependency areas, inviting staff from the intensive care unit, coronary care unit, and renal unit, as well as staff from the A and E.

The newly appointed staff nurses receive input from the staff nurse/bereavement counsellor on principles of caring for the suddenly bereaved relative as well as opportunities of reflecting on their own experience of caring for such relatives in A and E following a sudden death.

The newly appointed casualty doctors receive a lecture on caring for the dying patient and suddenly bereaved relative(s). Nurse learners are given a lecture on the same topic. They are encouraged to 'shadow' trained staff, to observe our way of managing sudden-death situations and gradually become involved in caring for relatives themselves, with opportunities later to reflect on and learn from such experiences.

8.5 CONCLUSIONS

Obviously, we have not arrived at an ideal way of caring for the dying patient and those suddenly bereaved, or supporting the A and E team who cares for them. The management I have outlined is not guaranteed to be fully implemented every time we have a sudden death, but it is what we do aim to provide for dying patients and those suddenly bereaved. Numbers of trained staff on-duty at any one time can vary greatly, and demands from patients in other areas of the department can be unpredictable due to the nature of the service we offer as an A and E Department. However, we feel caring for the dying patient and the suddenly bereaved relative(s) of patients who die in our department is an important and integral part of our role as Accident and Emergency nurses. As John Donne wrote in 1623:

No man is an Island entire of itself. Every man is a piece of the Continent, a part of the Main. Any man's death diminshes me because I am involved in Mankind. And therefore never send to know for whom the bell tolls, it tolls for thee.

EDITOR'S NOTES

This chapter must be read in conjunction with Chapter 5 on disaster and the references must apply to both. I have discussed at length with various groups, some of them disaster counsellors, the differences between sudden death of an individual, and multiple sudden deaths in a disaster. Problems of blame, responsibility and compensation may be major issues in disaster bereavement counselling. The main issues — grief, anguish and the realization that we may have little or no control over our lives — are the same for all.

My recent involvement with various groups of disaster workers has confirmed for me that emergency nurses have gained much experience and expertise in this area over many years. This sort of experience is difficult to gain or consolidate because it has the capacity to damage us or add to our emotional and psychological stature.

Susan McGuinness has, in a sensitive and methodical way, clarified a great deal about what we do. She also has new observations to make. I hope we can move away from the blinkered approach that we only learn by experiences.

REFERENCES

Ainsworth-Smith, I. and Speck, P. (1982) *Letting go: Care for the Dying and the Bereaved.* SPCK, London.

Bowling, A. (1983) The hospitalization of death: Should more people die at home? *Journal of Medical Ethics,* **9**, 158–61.

Elder, R.C. (1973) Social class and lay explanation of the etiology of arthritis. *Journal of Health Social Behaviour,* **14**, 24–38.

Forrest, G.C. (1983) *Oxford Study: Mourning the Loss of a Newborn Baby.* Bereavement Care, Cruse, Richmond, London.

Forrest, G.C., Standish, E., and Baum, J. D. (1982) Support after perinatal death: A study of support and counselling after perinatal bereavement. *British Medical Journal,* **285**, 1475–79.

Friedson, Elliot. (1961) *Patient's View of Medical Practice.* Russell Sage Foundation, New York.

Gerber, I. *et al.* (1975) *Grief Therapy to the Aged Bereaved. Bereavement: Its Psychological Aspects*, B. Schoenberg and I. Gerber (eds). Columbia University Press, New York.

Hoffman, M., Dorickers, S. and Hauser, M. (1978) The effects of nursing intervention on stress factors perceived by patients in a coronary care unit. *Heart and Lung*, **7** (September–October) no. 5, 804–9.

Le Poidevan, S. (1983) Model of adjustment to loss and change. Unpublished manuscript.

Lessa, W.A. and Vogt, E.Z. (eds). (1979) Reader in Comparative Religion, 4th edn. Harper and Row, New York.

Parkes, C.M. (1980) Bereavement counselling: Does it work? *British Medical Journal*, **2**, 3–6.

Parkes, C.M. (1981) *Bereavement: Studies of Grief in Adult Life*. Penguin Books, Harmondsworth, England.

Raphael, B. (1977) Preventive intervention with the recently bereaved. *Archives of General Psychiatry*, **34**, 1450–4.

Rudy, E.B. (1980) Patients' and spouses' causal explanation of a myocardial infarction. *Nursing Research*, **29**, 352–6.

Shapiro, E.I. (1983) Death and dying. *Journal of the Medical Society of New Jersey*, **80**(2), 110–13.

Thompson, J. (1983) Call Sister – stress in the Accident and Emergency Department. *Nursing Times*, 3 August, pp. 23–7.

Vachon, M.L.S. *et al.* (1980) A controlled study of self-help intervention for widows. *American Journal of Psychiatry*, **137**(ii), 1380–3.

Wilson, M. (1977) *Health is for People*. Darton, Longman and Todd, London.

Wright, B. (1980) Sudden death. *Nursing Mirror*, 13 November, pp. xxiv–xxix.

Young, G. (1980) In *Hospice and Health Care, Hospice: The Living Idea*, C. Saunders, D. Summers and N. Teller (eds). Edward Arnold, London.

FURTHER READING

Ashdown, M. (1985) Sudden death. *Nursing Mirror*, **161**, 18.

Cartwright, A., Hockey, L. and Anderson, J.L. (1973) *Life Before Death*. Routledge and Kegan Paul, London.

Dubin, W.R. and Sarnoff, J.R. (1983) Sudden unexpected death: intervention with survivors. *Annals of Emergency Medicine*, **15**, 86.

Parish, E., Holden, K.S. and Skiendzielewski, J.J. (1987) Emergency department experience with sudden death: A survey of survivors. *Annals of Emergency Medicine*, **16**, 7.

Rawlins, T. (1985) Survivors. *Nursing Times*, 27 November.

Taylor, H. (1984) *The hospice movement in Britain: Its role and future*. Centre for Policy on Ageing, London.

Wright, B. (1986) *Caring in crisis*. Churchill Livingstone, Edinburgh.

APPENDIX A

First research project (April 1983): Management of Suddenly Bereaved Relatives in the Accident and Emergency Department: Survey of available care and facilities.
To indicate your answer please (✔) tick the appropriate box.

1. Do you have a specific resuscitation area in your department?
   Yes ( )   No ( )

2. How many patients can be treated in this specific area at any one time?
   1–2 ( )   3–4 ( )   5–6 ( )   7–8 ( )   9–10 ( )

3. Where do those accompanying the critically ill patient admitted to the resuscitation area wait after being separated from the patient on admission?
   General waiting area   ( )
   Sister's office   ( )
   Doctor's office   ( )
   Staff coffee room   ( )
   Distressed relatives' room   ( )
   Other (please specify)   ( ) _____

4. What facilities are available to accompanying friends and relatives of critically ill patients waiting in the department?
   Public call box   ( )
   Private telephone   ( )
   (access to a telephone in a
   private room   ( )
   Vending machine (refreshments) ( )
   Other (please specify)   ( ) _____

5. Do you contact the hospital chaplain?
   Anglican
   ( ) Always ( ) Sometimes ( ) Never ( ) Only when requested
   Roman Catholic
   ( ) Always ( ) Sometimes ( ) Never ( ) Only when requested
   Other appropriate religious minister
   ( ) Always ( ) Sometimes ( ) Never ( ) Only when requested

6. Who usually tells the relatives and friends of the death?
   Nurse ( )   Doctor ( )   Both ( )

7. Do nurse learners accompany trained staff/doctors when caring for suddenly bereaved relatives?
   ( ) Always   ( ) Frequently   ( ) Infrequently   ( ) Never

8. Do you give any literature to the relatives when they leave the department after a sudden death?

( ) Yes   ( ) No

9. Do you only give verbal information to relatives about the implications (e.g. post-mortem)?

( ) Yes   ( ) No.

10. Who is responsible for looking after and liaising with the relatives when they are in the A and E?

Nursing officer	( )
Senior sister/charge nurse	( )
Trained member of staff	( )
Nurse learner allocated by senior sister/charge nurse/trained staff	( )
Nurse auxiliary allocated by senior sister/charge nurse/trained staff	( )

11. How many of the following personnel usually come into contact with the relatives and friends for any length of time that suddenly bereaved relatives are in the A and E?

Nursing officer	( )
Senior sister/charge nurse	( )
Trained member of nursing staff	( )
Nurse learner	( )
Nurse auxiliary	( )
Domestic staff	( )
Chaplain	( )
Social worker	( )
Police	( )
Ambulance crew	( )
Medical records officer	( )
Coroner's officers	( )
Nursing/General administration	( )
Volunteers from a bereavement-care service	( )

12. Is there any follow-up of relatives by the A and E once the relatives have left the department, e.g. telephoning them 24 hours after their bereavement?

( ) Yes   ( ) No

If Yes, please specify _____

13. Do you refer relatives for bereavement counselling?

( ) Yes   ( ) No

14. Would you be interested in receiving any literature that may result from this research project regarding the care of suddenly bereaved relatives in the A and E?

( ) Yes   ( ) No

If yes, please write your name and address below:

Name _____

Address _____

_____

Tel No _____ Ext _____

15.   Any other comments would be warmly welcomed.

Thank you for completing this questionnaire.

APPENDIX B

Second research project: The Nursing Management of Sudden Death in the Accident and Emergency Department

1. All information you give will be used for the benefit of research purposes only.
2. In order to keep the information anonymous, please insert your code number at the top, right-hand corner of each page.
3. There are no right or wrong answers.
4. If you would like a copy of the results of this research project, please place a tick in the box below.

☐

5. Please place tick in the appropriate box(es) unless otherwise indicated.

Thank you

1. How difficult is it for you to discuss sudden death with:
   a) your colleagues   Not difficult   ( )
                        Difficult   ( )
                        Very difficult   ( )
   b) senior staff   Not difficult   ( )
                        Difficult   ( )
                        Very difficult   ( )

2. Was this subject included in your orientation to the Accident and Emergency Department?
   Yes ( )   No ( )

3. By whom was this subject presented (e.g. doctor, sister, tutor)?
   Please state   _____

4. a) How do you feel when faced with the differing cultural attitudes and reactions to death and bereavement?
                              Able to cope   ( )
                              Unaffected   ( )
                              Anxious   ( )

   b) Which particular reactions do you find it most difficult to cope with, that should be covered in your orientation?

5. What preparation do you give to ancillary staff for being involved with the bereaved?
   Please state:

6. Do you feel you were adequately prepared to meet the needs of bereaved relatives following a sudden death in the A and E?

Yes ( )   No ( )

If no, please mention below any area you feel should have been included to meet your needs.

7. What do you consider the needs of bereaved relatives to be?

8. Please list the following nursing actions in order of priority in the event of a sudden death in the A and E.

( ) Custody of immediate personal effects of the deceased
( ) Arranging transport home for relatives
( ) Being prepared yourself to stay with the bereaved relatives according to their needs
( ) Notifying chaplain or other religious body
( ) Referral to bereavement service
( ) Provide refreshments and telephone to bereaved relatives
( ) Inform relatives of the death
( ) Facilitating the expression of feelings by relatives to the news of the death
( ) Providing literature for relatives, such as on funeral arrangements and legal implications of sudden death
( ) Viewing the body

Instructions: Please place a number inside bracket, e.g. (2), or write N/A for nursing actions not applicable to your A and E.

9. How did you feel when encountering sudden death for the first time in the A and E?

Please tick as appropriate

( ) angry	( ) stressed
( ) calm	( ) overwhelmed
( ) anxious	( ) helpless
( ) helpful	( ) controlled
( ) detached	( ) happy
( ) tearful	( ) unmoved
( ) frightened	( ) compassionate
( ) satisfied	( ) resentful
( ) guilty	( ) flippant
( ) unprepared	( ) frustrated

10. How do you feel now when encountering sudden death in the A and E?

( ) angry   ( ) stressed
( ) calm   ( ) overwhelmed
( ) anxious   ( ) helpless
( ) helpful   ( ) controlled
( ) detached   ( ) happy
( ) tearful   ( ) unmoved
( ) frightened   ( ) compassionate
( ) satisfied   ( ) resentful
( ) guilty   ( ) flippant
( ) unprepared   ( ) frustrated

11. Did your feelings affect the quality of your nursing actions?

Yes ( )   No ( )

If yes, how were they affected?

12. What opportunities are there for you to discuss your reactions following a sudden death during the rest of your day/night shift?

Always the opportunity   ( )
Frequently the opportunity   ( )
Infrequently the opportunity ( )
No opportunity available   ( )

13. What have you found to be most helpful in releasing emotional tension after a sudden death in the A and E? Please state.

14. What additional topics would be required in training to prepare you adequately for your role in working with patients and families in the A and E?

15. What specific communication difficulties do you have:

a) talking to dying patients

b) talking to relatives before a death?

c) talking to relatives after a death?

16. What reactions do you find most difficult to deal with:
a) in dying patients?

b) in relatives?

c) in yourself?

d) in colleagues?

17. Any other comments:

Thank you for completing this questionnaire

APPENDIX C

Susan Le Poidevan's model of counselling for adjustment to loss and change

The model of counselling is based on three skeletal structures which should be memorized:

i) Five time dimensions of adjustment
ii) Nine personality dimensions of adjustment
iii) Ten phases of the counselling process

The time dimensions and personality dimensions are integrated into the counselling process in interviewing, assessment, goal-setting and working through adjustments.

i) Five time dimensions of adjustment

Adjustment before death:	Adjustment after death:
Anticipation and prevention of avoidable problems	Progression from grief work to growth work

Phase 1: Adjustment to death as part of life
Phase 2: Adjustment to life-threatening illness from diagnosis
Phase 3: Crisis intervention at time of death
Phase 4: Adjustment after death 2–5 years
Phase 5: Adjustment to future stress and change

ii) *Nine personality dimensions of adjustment*

The counsellor must be able to get an overview of the whole person's unique adjustment to the event, bearing in mind long-term aims of healthy adjustment which guide the counselling process.

1. Intellectual - acceptance of the fact
              - implications of the loss
              - gradual process of realization and reconciliation
2. Psychological - formation of satisfactory identity and self-concept
              - self-esteem
              - defence and coping mechanisms
3. Spiritual - re-evaluation of philosophy
           - purpose and meaning of life
           - suffering and death
           - values and faith
4. Physical - minimization of stress related illness
5. Emotional - restoration of emotional balance
6. Sexual - coming to terms with one's own sexuality
          - satisfactory adjustment to changes in sexual behaviour
7. Behavioural - reorganization of routine and lifestyle with minimal disruption and stress
8. Social-cultural - reorganization of family and social structure
9. Practical - adaptation to practical demands of daily living

iii) *Ten phases of the counselling process*

1. Introduction - referral, finding out about counselling, contact
2. **Opening** - putting client at ease, establish rapport
3. **Interviewing** - getting the story
4. **Assessment** - summarizing themes, balancing strengths and problems
5. **Setting goals** - turning problems into action
6. Counselling decision and contact
7. Working through adjustments
8. Closing
9. Evaluating outcome
10. Feedback into practice

9

Encountering Hostility and Aggression

Bob Wright

The nurse in the Accident and Emergency Department will encounter all sorts of human conditions every day. The crisis of sudden illness and injury will produce intense and disruptive feelings. Some of these feelings will emerge as hostility and aggression.

We should begin by discussing the appropriateness of this response. If we feel that these feelings should be suppressed or totally controlled or that there is no place for them in our Department, we are being unrealistic. The outcome of hostile or aggressive feelings may be violent behaviour. We must work to prevent or suppress this response but the feelings of hostility and aggression are part of the human condition. We may respond in this way when overwhelmed with imminent loss or when we are threatened in some way. It may be the sudden spontaneous way in which we defend ourselves.

One reason we may react strongly against aggression is that it is the one component of our own emotional selves most would rather not confront. Any discussion of the problem is not just about what happens on the football terraces or to the underprivileged, but about ourselves. The problem can be social, political and personal. Discussion and exploration of the subject can produce strong feelings and emotions. As you follow the subject in this chapter, try to confront your own feelings honestly.

We have only to highlight two or three problems encountered daily in our work to focus on the way we encounter hostility and aggression.

- the battered wife whose husband arrives fearful she will want to report him to the police and desperate to get to her

- the loving sons and daughters of the elderly pedestrian knocked down by the drunken driver of a stolen car
- the forty-year-old man whose own business is just beginning to succeed, admitted to hospital with a myocardial infarction

We could go on with many more examples. Some of these situations have immediate and apparent components of aggression. For some people the helplessness, frustration and sadness may suddenly emerge as hostility. This surprises the person it emerges from as well as his loved ones. For the nurse working with them, it may suddenly produce fear and a need to defend oneself and the institution to which one is aligned. To encounter this response persistently and for long periods is stressful and potentially damaging. It is important therefore to consider the nature of hostility and aggression to remove some of our perplexity about it.

A greater understanding may remove some of our unrealistic expectations about hostility and perhaps remind us that these feelings are about us. This appraisal means we begin by examining our feelings about it and then move on to explore how we interact with the patient and his family.

9.1 THE NATURE OF VIOLENCE AND AGGRESSION

Ideas on what constitutes violence are full of confusion. The punch that makes contact is a violent act; the one that misses may be acceptable. Eysenck (1979) in outlining the various hypotheses that explain violence in present-day society, concludes that social and biological factors are responsible. He emphasizes the need to develop a conscience in children by conditioning them to control violent responses.

Others put forward the solution that improving our social environment or space will prevent disorder. Russell and Russell (1979) explain that studies of monkeys have demonstrated they are relaxed under spacious conditions while groups that are overcrowded quarrel, have brutal bosses and wound and kill each other. This led on to a discussion of over-stretched resources in crowded urban areas that produce aggression and violence.

Blood-spilling and other violence is often depicted alongside love, romance and adventure by the media. The manner in which these aspects are reconciled is highlighted by many as the cause of hostility, aggression and violence in society.

It could be argued that this short overview is pointless and that aggression will always be a part of our society and human nature. I think it is important that we look at some of the reasons behind our statistics of injured and violated people. We are in a good position to monitor trends and attitudes in society: to be confronted with our behaviour, its outcomes in society and the cost implications can only be healthy.

9.2 PREVENTING VIOLENT RESPONSES IN THE INDIVIDUAL

Emergency nurses have a wealth of information about peoples' behaviour. If I asked one of our experienced nurses which individuals from a waiting room full of people were likely to be disruptive, she would accurately choose one or two. Certain behaviours or responses can signal a person who is likely to erupt. We may witness this behaviour daily and be so flooded by the experience that we fail to act on the signals. The ensuing encounter may be difficult and put us at risk, so we may choose to avoid the confrontation.

The word 'confrontation' is loaded with difficult problems, but it does not have to be. Confrontation may allow some difficulty to emerge and be shared usefully. Signs that aggression and hostility are producing a situation that is getting out of control should be acted upon.

Whilst we may encounter these signs daily, I feel it is useful to set them down formally to increase our awareness of them and remind us of their importance. When the individual's usual coping mechanisms break down we begin to see signs that he is becoming restless, agitated and angry. We are witnessing the first signs of something that can culminate in destructive aggression.

9.3 SIGNALS THAT VIOLENCE IS DEVELOPING

Some identifiable signs of incipient violence:

1. There is a change in the individual's response to your role. You are no longer a person who can help him but someone who puts

obstacles in his way. You are preventing him from getting what he wants. What was previously perceived as helpful or useful now elicits little or no response.

2. He becomes restless and agitated, paces the floor, persistently looks into the treatment area, wrings his hands and looks at them.

3. Single acts of behaviour are provocative, attention-seeking or appear to demand punitive measures. This behaviour may take the form of using obscene words loudly or openly smoking in defiance of no-smoking signs.

4. He may demand immediate answers to difficult questions and enlist the help of others.

5. He begins to taunt you and attempts to bring you into disrepute. Sarcasm may be a strong component.

6. His voice becomes louder or he begins to shout.

7. You have difficulty in getting and keeping his attention and his ability to concentrate on what you say is poor.

8. Time becomes an important factor for you, the patient and his family. You have difficulty in focusing on your duties because of this and he has other important and pressing needs elsewhere.

9.4 RESPONDING TO THESE SIGNS

The nurse needs to respond to the individual and not to perform for the larger audience of the waiting area. Recognition of this removes from her some of the pressure to be seen to be winning any confrontation. Seeking audience approval is not a good reason to confront a hostile person if there is a choice. Instead, the nurse should invite the person to a private area or room, but not one that leaves her totally isolated. Nearby children, the elderly and others who are vulnerable will be grateful they are no longer at risk.

It will be useful for a hostile person to discharge some of the feelings you have witnessed in his behaviour, but not at the expense of others. Ask him to talk about the change in his attitude and behaviour and explain that you find it distressing to see him like this. If he relates better to someone else, allow him to do this. You are dealing with what is happening now, the immediate problem. If you take on his personality or lifestyle it may be such an enormous problem that you are tempted to give up immediately. When you have invested a lot of your time with this person it is easy to take remarks personally. Try to control your nonverbal and verbal responses to his behaviour. This may take the form of standing defiantly with your arms folded, which can be interpreted as being aggressive. When eye contact is maintained he knows he has your attention. A smile or a look around the room may be misinterpreted; standing too close may be invading his personal space. The intervention should have a definite focus with short-term, well-defined aims.

9.4.1 When violent behaviour occurs

When violent behaviour occurs the following actions are important to try to ensure safety and the best possible outcome for all concerned.

1. Call for help. This may sound obvious but it is often discovered later that it has not been done. Before the event sit down to discuss and organize formally how extra help can be found. It is useful to have a special number that the telephonists answer immediately as a signal to summon help. It will be necessary to discuss the management of these situations with your hospital security staff before the event. It may be necessary to call the police. What happens next will be decided after these different disciplines arrive.

2. Ask someone to remove other patients and relatives from danger. This may mean a hurried decision to change waiting or clinical areas but it is often easier than removing the violent patient.

3. Try not to get cornered. The layout of some departments provides rooms with limited access. Make a point of always using a room with through access when talking to someone who may be violent.

4. Avoid threats and raising your voice. Even though you may be physically struggling with the patient, keep talking. He may suddenly decide he will talk to someone. Often one person is singled out of the group with whom he wants to talk. Do not enter into a contract that leaves him alone with that person.

5. Restraining the patient should be done, if necessary, by using as many people as possible with one person per limb and two for the body. We do not want to hurt him. Avoid knees, feet or elbows being pressed into the body.

6. Do not enter into contracts you cannot keep. By glibly offering immunity from prosecution or the police you cause more problems. The hostile person will not trust you again and you may have to

encounter him another time. When he discovers promises were false it may provoke another aggressive outburst. The police would also be unhappy that you had spoken on their behalf.

After an act of violence has occurred and help has arrived, all concerned will now have to confer to decide on what to do next. If there is no clinical condition that demands hospital treatment the assailant must be removed from the premises. The police will decide then whether to release him or to keep him in custody. Later in this chapter we will look in more detail at how certain toxic conditions or organic illnesses may cause violence.

Whilst the police may have been involved in the initial management of a violent act, it may not be appropriate to enlist their continued help. Decisions about whether to detain, release or sedate a patient are often difficult ones. If the patient has a serious head injury, we do not want to compromise our evaluation of his conscious level. However, it may be in his and everyone else's interest to sedate him despite this clinical condition.

Before concluding this section on the management of a violent incident, I want to make the following points. Some nurses will have some anxiety about detaining a patient against his will during, or after, a violent incident. The legal position is often helped by the presence of the police. In Britain a psychiatric nurse may detain a patient for six hours under the 1983 Mental Health Act. This may be one of the advantages of having a psychiatric nurse in the A and E Department. A court will treat sympathetically nurses or other persons who detain a person in hospital against his will if they acted in good faith. It is unlikely a case such as this would get to the courtroom. Nurses from North America may wonder why I have not discussed the use of mechanical restraint. Wrist and ankle straps and body belts may be incorporated into trolleys to restrain a patient. During a working visit to the US I witnessed these being used. The only advantage I could see was that it allowed the many personnel involved to be released more quickly. If resources are scarce this is important. I believe human involvement with the violent person is more important, especially if it is not to be seen as punitive.

9.5 USEFUL DRUGS

It may be necessary to use pharmaceutical means to control violence. Drugs that sedate or tranquillize will be suggested here. If the violence is associated with a hypoglycaemic attack, a 50% dextrose solution given intravenously may be effective, and this should be kept available. Appropriate treatment should also be available to treat other conditions that may produce violence, such as epilepsy. Many medical and surgical conditions may produce a violent response and it is beyond the scope of this chapter to explore all of these.

The following drugs have been found useful in the management of violence associated with psychiatric illness and other states of acutely disturbed behaviour.

9.5.1 Chlorpromazine

Chlorpromazine is the most commonly used drug in the control of psychotic hostility. It can be given by deep intramuscular injection or orally in the form of syrup or tablets. Tablets may be secreted in the mouth by the more suspicious patient. However, a 50–100 mg intramuscular injection will make the patient drowsy within 30 minutes. If necessary, and depending on the size of the patient, this can be repeated after one to two hours. The drug is less well tolerated by the elderly as it can produce marked hypotension, and if used in these patients an initial dose of 25 mg may be better tolerated.

All phenothiazine drugs potentiate the effects of barbiturates and alcohol. Care must be exercised when dealing with violent patients whose outburst was precipitated by either of these.

9.5.2 Haloperidol

In mania and hypomania, Haloperidol can be used in dosages sufficient to control aggressive behaviour without the risk of hypotension encountered with phenothiazines. Haloperidol is a butyrophenone that has properties and side-effects similar to phenothiazines, but a reduced risk of hypotension. It can be given orally in tablet or liquid form or by intramuscular or intravenous injection. It has a prolonged action which means that a dose of 5–10 mg may last for 24 hours.

Both Chlorpromazine and Haloperidol may produce a dystonic reaction in some patients. This is shown by rigidity, a shuffling gait and protruding tongue which will produce fear and anxiety in an already distressed patient. Another side-effect may be an occular-gyric crisis in which the occulo-motor nerves of the eyes are affected and the patient can only look upwards.

A 10 mg intramuscular injection of Procyclidine will remove the unwanted occular-gyric side-effect. It may also be administered slowly by intravenous infusion.

Our immediate problem, and the focus of this chapter, is the management of a violent episode. It is nevertheless worth remembering that once drugs are administered, they will sedate the patient and suppress symptoms. This may produce a problem when a psychiatrist needs evidence to detain a patient compulsorily in a psychiatric hospital. If one or two people need evidence of psychiatric disorder to detain the patient, the administration of drugs may impede this.

9.5.3 Benzodiazepines

It has long been recognized that, far from reducing hostility, drugs in the benzodiazepine group may facilitate its emergence. Gardos *et al.* (1968) reported the effects of Chlordiazepoxide, Diazepam and Oxazepam on a group of student volunteers. Whilst the drugs reduced anxiety, the volunteers displayed an increase in overtly hostile and aggressive behaviour. This is of particular significance in the management of the aggressive self-poisoning patient whose behaviour may be the direct result of the drugs prescribed for him to reduce his anxiety.

Diazepam is of value in controlling the acutely disturbed behaviour that may be associated with epilepsy. The intravenous administration of 5–10 mg will usually control aggressive behaviour in these patients.

9.6 SPECIAL PROBLEMS

The following conditions create special problems that merit some individual consideration.

9.6.1 Organic Reactions

The main clinical features in patients with organic reactions are:

(a) Confusion. The patient becomes bewildered and perplexed by what seems to him to be a strange and meaningless series of events. This leads to a state of:
(b) Disorientation. He is unable to give details of the correct date, day or time of year. He will have difficulty with the identity and roles of the health care staff who surround him. Some of these, such as the nurse in uniform, will have a visually clearly definable role.
(c) Fear and apprehension. These feelings can lead to acute panic attacks which themselves can result in outbursts of violent behaviour.
(d) Hallucinations. These may be particularly unpleasant and terrifying. Some patients see hordes of insects coming towards them or crawling over their skin. Nurses talking outside the room may be misinterpreted as being hostile and plotting to kill the patient.
(e) Agitation and restlessness. Not surprisingly, patients may become violent in their attempts to protect themselves or escape.

Whilst we cannot go into great detail on all of these conditions, Table 9.1 gives us some idea about the sorts of conditions we should bear in mind. Some of the conditions listed here are a timely reminder that we can make quick but inaccurate decisions or assumptions about precipitating factors surrounding aggression and hostility to the detriment of the patient's well-being.

Table 9.1 Some Organic Causes of Aggression

Infection: Dehydration
Intoxication: Alcohol, drugs
Cardiovascular disease: Hypoxia
Respiratory disturbance: Hypoxia
Vitamin deficiency: Chronic alcoholism, chronic illness
Post-operative conditions: Shock, anaesthesia
Metabolic disorder: Diabetes, uraemia
Endocrine disorder: Thyrotoxicosis, puerperal
Head injury

Source: Compiled by the author

9.6.2 The elderly

Aggression in the elderly is a problem most nurses find very distressing. The confused, frail and frightened elderly patient who is attempting to leave but is obviously at risk produces a terrible dilemma. To restrain the patient physically and further damage our rapport with her is upsetting and makes us feel bad about ourselves. The confusion that hospital admission produces may mean that these patients are not always given the attention that they deserve or that they are not taken seriously. Many conditions in the elderly lead to confusion and aggression and make a problem-solving approach not at all straightforward or easy. The causes of confusion listed by Faulkner (1985) seem to me to be a useful approach. In addition to the organic causes mentioned above, she goes on to list such psychosocial causes as changes in environment, isolation and bereavement trauma.

The special problem of sedating elderly patients is discussed above in the section on useful drugs.

9.6.3 Crisis

The accessibility of the Accident and Emergency Department's 24-hour service means that many people experiencing one of life's crises find themselves in that Department. Whilst some patients will have injury or illness associated with the crisis, others will be present for no other reason than the crisis, which is the reason for their feeling ill. Berrios (1982) in his paper on psychiatric emergencies found that 30-40% of these emergencies seen in the Accident and Emergency Department were behavioural disturbances resulting from a breakdown in family communications.

He also suggested that doctors should be able to identify the social nature of these emergencies and consult relatives and friends to obtain a comprehensive history. This is time-consuming and in my view an unnecessary use of the doctor's time. A study I undertook in the US demonstrated that psychiatric nurses were able to intervene quite adequately and refer patients to the appropriate agency (Wright 1985). I am firmly of the opinion that nurses in Accident and Emergency need to gain further skills in crisis intervention so that they can offer total care of the patient with his illness or injury. Attempting to separate the emotional crisis from the patient can produce all sorts of problems. A framework within which to work and a knowledge of the process is described in my study of this aspect of emergency nursing (Wright 1986).

9.6.4 Self-poisoning

Self-poisoning patients can make up a large proportion of our medical admissions. A problem in the immediate management is to treat assertively the poisoning aspect of the patient's condition without losing focus on the emotional crisis that precipitated the episode. To ask the patient to save his emotional problems until a later stage in the proceedings when a specialist worker will be available may be asking the impossible. To fail to respond to or accept and hear the feelings of the patient may be seen as devaluing him.

Many patients who are seen in the Emergency Department after a self-poisoning act are angry. We must examine our care of these patients thoroughly and ask ourselves if our approach to the patient is fragmented. There are many other reasons why the patient feels hostile and acts aggressively. They may well feel stupid at having failed to kill themselves and angry at their own inadequacy. The lowering of self-esteem which they experience leads to a feeling that they do not deserve to succeed in a relationship. The feelings associated with this predicament are overwhelmingly painful and distressing. It may be too much to cope with and too much of a burden. A sudden, immense desire to escape this problem may result in impulsive and desperate attempts to leave.

It can also be difficult to own up to such feelings and the patient may well angrily displace them onto the nurse. It is not surprising that there are some strong feelings of anger and aggression in the self-poisoning patient. Aggression turned inwardly on oneself may also result in an act of self-mutilation.

9.6.5 Self-mutilation

It is difficult to separate patients with self-mutilation from the one described in the next section as having a personality disorder. Acts of self-mutilation deserve a special mention despite this close association because of the strong component of aggression and the potential for violence. The cutting of wrists or arms are the most common means and sites of injury and may precipitate admission. It must not be assumed that the act of self-mutilation is now over. If the patient feels he is being treated in any way differently or with contempt, then he may repeat the act.

After a rapport has been established it is advisable to ask if any more razor blades or the knife used for self-injury can be handed to the staff. When a patient cuts himself dramatically in front of staff or others the staff may respond with fear and revulsion. These feelings may produce unthinking and hazardous responses from the staff. Sudden attempts to remove weapons may leave staff cornered and injured or even occasionally in a hostage situation. It is difficult to keep calm and respond in a controlled way when witnessing acts of self-mutilation, but it is important that you do so.

This sort of histrionic behaviour is usually found in patients who can best be described as having a personality disorder. It must also be remembered that some depressive patients, especially adolescents, respond in this way. We will next consider the management of these patients who fit loosely into the category of personality disorder.

9.6.6 Personality disorders

The way we interact with others in our personal relationships, occupations, social settings and in stressful situations depends to a large extent on our personality. The traits in our personalities are developed over a lifetime. When these traits persistently impair the patient's social and occupational functioning or cause continuing emotional distress, a personality disorder is possibly present.

In talking to the patient you may well elicit some history of job failure, marital problems or irresponsible or illegal behaviour that has led to a prison record. The reckless and impulsive behaviour that led to the individual's hospitalization may still be apparent in his interaction with you. Such patients antagonize you, the staff, because they respond aggressively to your efforts to help them, they demand immediate attention and it is difficult to remain well-motivated towards helping them.

It is interesting that they generate a powerful negative reaction amongst the staff and this gut feeling of staff is a good indication of the patient's damaged personality. We must acknowledge how useful an indicator this response is, but not respond in a negative way. This is the difficult bit. To remain nonjudgemental whilst acknowledging our feelings is a skill we need to work on.

Patients with personality disorders are notoriously difficult to handle, and in the long term, difficult to treat. They have become comfortable with periods of disruption and crisis in their lives and have come to expect them. It is therefore very rewarding when we can use the immediate situation effectively to help them to get some help from the appropriate agency or gain some insight into what is happening. If we manage to treat the injury or illness without a great deal of disruption, something has been achieved. It reminds them that this is possible in the long term and that someone cares about them.

We will be disappointed if we set unrealistic goals and expect major change in the patient during our limited interactions with him. We should nevertheless continue in our efforts to promote health and rehabilitation. The day we give patients up as totally hopeless may be the day we have to re-examine our motivation and skills.

9.6.7 The psychiatric patient

Acutely psychotic behaviour, as exhibited by schizophrenics or manic depressive psychotics, accounts for many of the admissions to the A and E Department. The patient may develop delusions or hallucinations and may behave in a bizarre way or express strange ideas. The difficulty in making contact on a meaningful level with this patient may be a good indication of a schizophrenic illness. You will feel strongly the strange and bizarre thoughts of the patient as they are usually well communicated. The overtly grandiose and euphoric mood of the hypomanic patient, his hyperactivity and happiness, swinging sometimes to sadness, will on the other hand be easy to identify with. These patients are popular and amusing and nurses initially find them interesting. This contrasts strongly with the uneasy and strained interactions we have with schizophrenics. Both illnesses produce unpredictable episodes of aggression and violence and other powerful outpourings of hostility.

The immediate management of the patient by the psychiatrist may be medication and compulsory detention. Whilst compulsory detention is necessary, it produces much hostility. The patient also has a right to be fully aware of this detention and under what statutes it is being enforced. Before this information is given it is worth having some extra help available.

It is not within the scope of this chapter to look in detail at psychiatric illness. The shift of resources to community care and the closing down of large psychiatric hospitals will produce many more psychiatric emergencies for A and E Departments. For this reason we need much more in-service training for staff on psychiatric illness.

The list of special problems associated with physiological and psychological conditions could be endless. The seven areas examined above outline some common problems. Our skill and curiosity about why patients respond in hostile and aggressive ways will help us to deal with other medical conditions that produce this response. The psychosocial aspects of patient care are also an important factor.

9.7 ORGANIZATIONAL FACTORS THAT CONTRIBUTE TO HOSTILITY

The following factors contribute to hostility and can be avoided.

1. *Waiting*. Priorities in the A and E Department change unexpectedly. Life-threatening problems may suddenly occur simultaneously and all resources have to be directed to that area of care. We must look seriously at ways of making the waiting area more pleasant, with diversions from waiting time. Piped-in music, videos, books, magazines and toys for children in a special play area are just some ideas that could be used to achieve this. Providing up-to-date information to patients about why they are having to wait will dissipate some of their frustration.

2. *Separation of the patient from his family*. The doctor needs to examine the patient in privacy where there can be a frank and total exchange of information. Relatives often resent this. When a large number of relatives are present it is difficult to decide who should stay with the patient and it may be easier just to exclude them all. Explain to them why they are being separated from the patient. If treatment, investigations or procedures are prolonged, tell the relatives why they are waiting. If at all possible, get to know who the relatives are and where they are waiting.

3. *Pain*. Hostility is often a response to pain. Pain increases when patients are kept waiting for long periods or when they are isolated.

4. *Noise*. This adds to the general feeling of chaos and disorder. It attacks the senses and may produce a desire to escape from it.

5. *Lack of understanding of the system.* Some Departments have a leaflet that describes the different priorities given to different conditions. It goes on to explain why patients may not be seen in chronological order. It may also explain that, unbeknownst to one patient, another may be being admitted with serious or life-threatening injuries and will therefore be given priority. Keeping people informed may save a lot of time and effort and a handout given to the patient or relative on arrival is a way of doing this.

6. *Failure to act on behavioural signals.* The organization must continually keep staff aware and updated in skills of intervention and communication. This not only prevents violence but also averts burnout by confronting staff with knowledge of their performance and keeps them well-motivated.

7. *Failure to share decisions with the patient or family.* If decisions are taken by others that are important to you and your life, it is obvious that you will want to be involved. However, it remains a fact that we persistently fail to involve the patient or relatives in our plans for his treatment and care. This will produce anger and can be avoided.

8. *Prejudice.* Most of us have some prejudice about behaviour, race, colour or creed. It is essential that we confront each other and ourselves with this prejudice. How it affects our responses, behaviour and care of the patient is an area that we need to explore.

9. *Delay in answering enquiries.* In large and busy Departments, patients can be in any of several areas or may be referred to other Departments. Anxious waiting relatives will not understand the complexities of this and may become agitated at our lack of awareness of where their loved one is. I believe we have not spent enough time in examining better ways of locating patients. We need some business expertise to help us map the movement of patients so that we can trace and eventually locate them quickly when their relatives arrive.

These are just a few of the organizational factors within the Emergency Department that can be powerful components in producing an aggressive and violent response. We are often resistant to changes within the organization because we are comfortable and safe working within the parameters of the status quo. This can be so even when we know it militates against good patient care because change can be too disruptive to us. It also takes a tremendous amount of persuasion and motivation to facilitate change.

9.8 EVALUATION OF INCIDENTS OF VIOLENCE

It is absolutely essential to maintain good records of violent incidents, not just for legal reasons but also to improve our practice. In our regular evaluation of these incidents we may highlight organizational problems that contribute to violence. We may also identify staff who show prejudice or who lack certain skills. It may become apparent that certain staff members are always the ones to intervene in these incidents because others avoid them. There will be much useful evidence that we may need in order to increase staffing levels, engage more security staff or monitor disturbing social changes. It is important to remember that what happens in the A and E Department often reflects what is going on in the outside world. This is one aspect of our work of which we may not wish to be reminded.

The emergency management of the aggressive and hostile patient in the A and E Department is very stressful. There are many other demands being made on the nurse, who is often under the watchful eye of many other people. This includes colleagues, the patients and the public. The issues involved produce strong feelings and it is easy for those on the periphery to become involved. Such a situation has all the potential for becoming too big and difficult to handle. It produces abject fear and distress and, unfortunately, injury. We must therefore have good policies, good assessment of the patient's clinical condition and some anticipation of his emotional needs. The skillful preparation of staff for this work is vital together with a good continuing education programme.

Aggression can be a positive emotion. Let us aim to keep it that way.

EDITOR'S NOTES

Since writing this chapter I have been a member of a government working party investigating more effective ways of preventing violence and protecting staff. Two reports studied by this committee are at the end of my Further Reading list.

Further literature relevant to the subject and training material for teaching staff about some of the issues, are available in *Violence in the National Health Service* by Ron Wiener and Sue Kilroe. This booklet and video are available from the Faculty Office, Faculty of Health Sciences and Social Studies, Leeds Polytechnic, Calverley Street, Leeds LS1 3HE, England. This is a must for every A and E Department and nursing school library.

REFERENCES

Berrios, E.E. (1982) Psychiatric emergencies. *Hospital Update*, **8**, 3.
Eysenck, H.J. (1979) The origin of violence. *Journal of Medical Ethics*, **5**, 105–7.
Faulkner, A. (1985) *Nursing: A Creative Approach*. Balliere Tindall, London.
Gardos, E., Dimasicio, A., Salzman, C. and Shader, R.I. (1968) Differential actions of Chlordiazepoxide and Oxazepam on hostility. *Archives of General Psychiatry*, **18**, 00–00.
Russell, C. and Russell, W.M.S. (1979) The natural history of violence. *Journal of Medical Ethics*, **5**, 108–17.
Wright, B. (1985) Psychiatric nurse clinicians in emergency areas. In *Recent Advances in Psychiatric Nursing*, A.J. Altshul (ed.). Churchill Livingstone, Edinburgh.
Wright, B. (1986) *Caring in Crisis – A Handbook of Intervention Skills for Nurses*. Churchill Livingstone, Edinburgh.

FURTHER READING

Brown, C.G. (1982) The alcohol withdrawal syndrome. *Annals of Emergency Medicine*, **11**, 276–80.
Burnard, P. (1987) Counselling: basic principles in nursing. *The Professional Nurse*, **2**, 9.
Department of Health and Social Security (1987) *Violence to Staff*. DHSS Branch C52A, Elephant and Castle, London.
Gilmore, G.M. (1986) Behavioural management of the acutely intoxicated patient in the emergency department. *Journal of Emergency Nursing*, **12**, 1.
Health and Safety Commission (1987) *Violence to Staff in the Health Services*. Health Services Advisory Committee, HMSO, London.

Index